Niamh Orbinski is a Nutritionist, Certified Intuitive Eating Counselor and Yoga Teacher. She runs a weight-inclusive, virtual nutrition practice specializing in intuitive eating, disordered eating and body image. Her day-to-day involves working with people one-on-one and through her programmes to help them leave dieting behind and rebuild a healthier relationship with food, movement and body image. Her work is HAES (Health At Every Size) aligned, meaning that she encourages health-promoting behaviours, regardless of their outcome on weight. She is a proud Carlow woman but these days calls Dublin home. This is her first book.

No Apologies

Ditch Diet Culture and Rebuild Your Relationship with Food

Niamh Orbinski

HarperCollins*Ireland*

HarperCollins*Ireland*
Macken House,
39/40 Mayor Street Upper,
Dublin 1
D01 C9W8
Ireland

a division of
HarperCollins*Publishers*
1 London Bridge Street,
London SE1 9GF
United Kingdom

www.harpercollins.co.uk

First published by HarperCollins*Ireland* in 2023
1

A catalogue record for this book is available from the British Library.

ISBN: 978-0-00-856720-0

Set in Capitana by Palimpsest Book Production Ltd, Falkirk, Stirlingshire

Printed and bound in the UK using
100% Renewable Electricity by CPI Group (UK) Ltd

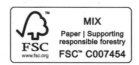

For all my amazing past, present and future clients who have chosen and trusted me to be a part of their precious journey of rebuilding their relationship with food and their body. Thank you for doing the work, which allows me to do mine and live my purpose.

Contents

Preface

How did we get here? How did I come to feel the need to write a book called *No Apologies*? Well, let me ask you. How is your relationship with food? Is it easy, effortless, and stress-free or is it stress-inducing and difficult? If you picked up this book, I'm guessing the latter. We live in a world that prioritises thinness over all else, for all genders, but especially for women. We grow up with media that paint a picture that in order to be happy you need to be thin. If you're not thin, you should be actively pursuing thinness. And if you are thin, you must desperately maintain it at all costs. What is this all about and where did it come from? A male friend asked me one day, 'Why do women wear fake tan?' I answered, 'Do you want the short answer or the long answer?' The same applies here. There are many socio-cultural and historical reasons why we find ourselves in this world obsessed with thinness and it has a lot to do with diet culture. If we are taught we need to be thin, and we're not thin, then there's a perceived problem that requires a solution. Diet culture provides us with that solution. It doesn't just sell diets, it sells a dream. Happiness, success, love, desirability — apparently thinness gets you all of these things and more! But at what cost? If my clients' stories are anything to go by, I'd say a lot. I'm sure you know people who have been dieting for decades but are larger than they've ever been. Perhaps you're one of those people. If so, I'm here to tell you this is not your fault, despite what you've been told or led to believe. Diet culture is at fault. It teaches us to feel as though we are not enough, that we have to apologize for ourselves or that we need to make ourselves smaller.

Before you can pursue true health, you need to have a healthy relationship with food, which, unfortunately, for many people, is not the case. To begin rebuilding a healthy relationship with food and body image, we must first understand why so many of us have an unhealthy relationship with food in the first place. You weren't born hating your body or worrying about food. It's a learnt behaviour. You will need to dissect the beliefs that maintain these behaviours and remove those that do not serve you. Only then will you be free to pursue health and treat your body like the magnificent container that it is. The one that carries you through life and allows you to experience the great moments and the small moments. I want that so much for you, so you can live a healthy, happy and fulfilled life for as long as possible. None of us has complete control over our health, no matter our size, but reading this book and implementing the steps outlined within will support you in accepting and nourishing the body that you have right now.

Every word written in this book has been inspired by the incredible people I have counselled over the years toward healthier relationships with food and their bodies. The stories I have heard have sometimes broken my heart, but the breakthroughs I have witnessed have made me cry with pride at the incredible resilience and strength of the human spirit. I am so honoured and privileged to do this work every day, and I am so grateful to everyone who has put their trust in me to guide them. I don't take even one client for granted and am consistently fascinated by every person sitting in front of me, who has shared their stories, innermost thoughts, emotions, doubts, wins, and challenges with me. It may be a cliché, but this book would not exist without you. Thank you to you all, and thank you, dear reader, for picking up this book. I hope it allows you and as many people as possible, no matter your difficulties or privileges, to experience your own version of food freedom and live your life unapologetically. I am cheering you on always.

Introduction

'Raise your hand if you've *never* been on a diet.'

It was 2021. I was standing at the front of a room, about to give a presentation to a crowd of people on intuitive eating and our relationship with food. This was the first request I made of them, the words in capital letters on a large screen in front. Can you guess how many people raised their hands?

Two. Just two.

Dieting, in some form, is so normalised that in a large crowd of people a minuscule percentage of them had never embarked on one. The urge to diet usually comes from a place of lack. From a feeling that you are not good enough as you are and that you need to fix or change some part of yourself. And it's not without cost for a lot of people who follow that urge. That cost is a healthy relationship with food. If you were to explain your relationship with food in one word, what would it be? If you've picked up this book, I'm guessing that it's none of the following:

- ☐ Free
- ☐ Easy
- ☐ Effortless
- ☐ Non-consuming

The relationship you have with food and your body is one of the most intimate relationships you will ever have. It has the power to dictate whether you survive or thrive in life. The health of this relationship can affect all other relationships in your life and it needs to be nurtured, just like any other relationship.

Humans are fragile creatures; we need to be fed and watered multiple times a day just to stay alive. Every day, we make an estimated 200 food-related decisions.[1] How crazy is that when you think about it? Those decisions can be easy and effortless, or they can be hard work. There's no way around it: you will have to feed yourself daily for the rest of your life. There is so much information out there about what we 'should' and 'should not' eat, but most of these conversations don't include the importance of how we feel around food and the impact this can have on our health and well-being. The relationship you have with food and your body can be positive, free, and easy, or it can be damaging, restrained, and complex. If you'd like to have the former, then you're in the right place. I work with people every day who feel the latter. Their relationship with food and body image often feels:

- ☐ Controlled
- ☐ Uneasy

☐ Difficult

☐ All-consuming

You might be thinking, 'Am I bad enough to need this book?' but we have all been affected, to some degree or another, by the messages from diet culture that encourage us to abandon our bodies. To prioritise external cues over internal ones and to disconnect from our inner wisdom. To constantly feel that our bodies are not good enough and that they need to be fixed or changed. Your body is your home. It's the only home you'll ever have and one to which only you can gain access. You are the expert of your own body. Only you know what you are feeling at any given moment. Only you know how hungry or full you are. Only you know what foods will satisfy you and what won't. This means that only you can know what exactly it is you need at any given moment. What a gift to know that you have everything you need within.

But sometimes we just need a little help and guidance to unlock it. That's where this book comes in. No matter how little or how much you struggle with your relationship with food, this book aims to help you. My hope is that it will support you in learning how to look after yourself from a compassionate non-diet lens, free from the constraints of diet culture. It takes into account your emotional and mental health, not just your physical health. Let's get started.

Who Is This Book For?

Is your relationship with food or body image holding you back from fully living your 'one wild and precious life'? Does it take up more time and energy than you'd like it to? What if I told you that eating could be easy and effortless? That it's possible to create a life full of health and free from food or body image obsession?

You might not believe me if you've struggled with food, weight, or implementing sustainable, healthy habits. Disordered eating rates in women are estimated to be between 50 per cent and 75 per cent.[2] If you're a man, thank you for picking up this book and please don't stop reading: this book is for you too. Unfortunately, male data is lacking, but that doesn't mean that men don't struggle.

Given that high number, I guarantee there are more than a few people you know who struggle with this too. The problem? They may not know it. Disordered eating is often disguised because it's seen as normal. That family member who's always on a diet and struggles with yo-yoing weight, that conversation over dinner with a friend that turned to feelings of guilt after having three courses, or meeting a buddy in the gym on a Monday evening who said they have to 'work off' their over-indulgence at the weekend. Despite their problematic nature, these are all examples of disordered eating that are often encouraged in our culture. In a world where we are overstimulated and have, one might say, too much information at the tips of our fingers, we still struggle to implement healthy habits and stick to them. We are a world obsessed with weight, yet the 'obesity epidemic' rages on. Many people believe it's their fault and blame themselves. But more information is often not what's needed — a connection to our own body and inner wisdom is. This book aims to change that by guiding you back to your inherent inner wisdom so that you can live a life full of health and free from food and body obsession. This book is for you, your mother, father, sister, brother, friends, and work colleagues. It's for anyone who would like to improve their health and get back into the driver's seat of their own life, reuniting with the expert within.

What Is (and Isn't) a Healthy Relationship with Food?

We all have a relationship with food and it has developed throughout our lives. Like any relationship in life, sometimes it can take a bashing and you might need to work on it to allow it to flourish and enhance your life, rather than take energy away from you.

Imagine your brain is a pie chart. Think about how much of your brain space each day is taken up thinking about food or your body. Can you put a percentage on it? What would that be? We all think about food on a daily basis. We have to — I mean, it keeps us alive, right? Some normal thoughts are:

- ☐ What's in the fridge?

- ☐ Do I need to go shopping?

- ☐ Do I need to prepare food this week to support a busy schedule?

- ☐ Would I like to try a new recipe?

- ☐ Do I need to add anything to my diet to make my body feel better — fibre, carbs, vegetables, water, and so on?

This, of course, will take up some space, and if you're working on a health goal and using nutrition to get there, the amount of space allocated to it may fluctuate, but in general, it shouldn't take up any more than 10 to 30 per cent. When I ask my clients this question, the average answer I receive is anywhere from 50 to 90 per cent. It's seen as normal to think and talk about food and your weight all of the time. This is precisely the issue. Since conversations around food and weight are so common, many people have an unhealthy relationship with food but don't realise it. Why would you when how you feel and behave around food is emulated by your family, your friends, and your colleagues? However, it's completely possible to get this percentage down. A client I recently finished up working with originally answered 90 per cent to this question. Now, her answer is 30 per cent. So if you feel preoccupied with food and your body image, I hope this gives you hope for the future.

It's important to note that having an unhealthy relationship with food doesn't mean that you have an eating disorder, but for some people, it may progress into an eating disorder if it's not treated. This book is not explicitly written for people with an eating disorder (although it should help, alongside treatment). It's written for anyone who identifies with the below components of an unhealthy relationship with food:

- ☐ Do you wake up thinking about food and go to bed thinking about food?

- ☐ Do you feel guilt or shame around food?

- ☐ Do you feel like you have to cut certain foods out of your diet?

☐ Is your diet inflexible, rather than flexible?

☐ Is your diet lacking in a wide variety of foods?

☐ Do you feel out of control around food, or do you binge or overeat when you get access to restricted foods or foods you think are bad?

☐ Do you feel addicted to food?

☐ Are you always on some kind of diet or lifestyle plan that dictates what, when, and how much to eat?

☐ Do you feel like you need to micromanage your diet and lifestyle to control your weight?

If you identify with any of these things, please know that it's completely possible to rebuild your relationship with food. I know because I've helped and seen hundreds of people do it. You are not a lost cause.

Ellyn Satter is a highly influential dietician and psychotherapist who has had a clinical career in this area for over forty years and is considered an internationally recognized authority on eating and feeding. She coined the components of 'normal eating' in 1983, which still ring true today. Here are some examples of a healthy relationship with food, taken from her work, to give you an idea of what you can look forward to.[3]

Normal eating is going to the table hungry and eating until you are satisfied.

It is being able to choose the food you like and eat it and truly get enough of it — not just stopping eating because you think you should.

It is being able to give some thought to your food selection so you get nutritious food, but not being so wary and restrictive that you miss out on enjoyable food.

It is giving yourself permission to eat sometimes because you are happy, sad, or bored, or just because it feels good.

It is mostly three meals a day, or four or five, or it can be choosing to munch along the way.

It is leaving some cookies on the plate because you know you can have some again tomorrow, or it is eating more now because they taste so wonderful.

It is overeating at times, feeling stuffed and uncomfortable.

And it can be undereating at times and wishing you had more.

It is trusting your body to make up for your mistakes in eating.

It takes up some of your time and attention, but keeps its place as only one important area of your life.

In short, normal eating is flexible. It varies in response to your hunger, your schedule, your proximity to food, and your feelings. External rules often govern an unhealthy relationship with food. A healthy relationship with food relies on your internal cues. You drive the bus, not diet culture. It is trusting your body's wisdom and allowing it to be your guide. You have everything you need within. But most people are in some way disconnected from this inner wisdom. Rebuilding your relationship with food is, in a way, a sort of coming home to your own body.

I have expanded on this in the free quiz and video training in the tools that accompany this book. Here, you'll be able to assess your own eating behaviours, so make sure you navigate to my website nutritionwithniamh.com to delve a little deeper into your own relationship with food. Do it right now, before you forget — it will only take a few minutes to complete the quiz and will set you up nicely for the rest of the book.

What Is Disordered Eating?

Our eating behaviours lie on a continuum between intuitive eating and clinical eating disorders. Between these two lies disordered eating. Disordered eating is a term used to describe a range of irregular eating behaviours that may not warrant a diagnosis of a specific eating disorder. It is a descriptive phrase, not a diagnosis. If someone is struggling with disordered eating, it doesn't mean they automatically have an eating disorder. For some people it may, but they are usually in the minority. Most of the people that I work with in my practice typically lie somewhere In the middle of this continuum. The place you find yourself on the spectrum Is not static, it is fluid, and it's possible to flow up and down this spectrum. This means that it's possible to move back towards intuitive eating, otherwise known as normal or healthy eating, or towards clinical eating disorders. I work with people to bring them closer to their intuitive eater and to prevent them from progressing on to a clinical eating disorder.

Having a healthy relationship with food is something we all deserve, but the eating patterns that we may consider normal are anything but. These behaviours may actually be promoted in order to lose weight or maintain a certain shape — think restricting from Monday to Friday or abstaining from certain foods because they induce guilt or shame. Disordered eating behaviours can occur as a symptom of diet backlash — the cumulative side effects of dieting. These can be short term or chronic, depending on how long a person has been dieting. It may be just one side effect or several.

You may spend an awful lot of time each day thinking about the type of food you eat or experience a lot of guilt and shame when you eat certain foods, but because these behaviours don't meet the criteria for an eating disorder, you're left feeling like it's not a problem. And sure, everyone thinks like this, right? That might be the case, but it doesn't mean that it's a healthy way to approach food. If it's distressing you, you deserve to seek help. Period. Disordered eating behaviours deserve attention and treatment, as they may turn into more problematic eating disorders if they don't receive some TLC. Unlike eating disorders, there isn't a classification of symptoms that warrant a diagnosis; however, there are many behaviours that can fall into this category. Some of these are taken from the Eat Right website, run by the Academy of Nutrition and Dietetics in the US.[4]

Signs and symptoms of disordered eating may include, but are not limited to:

☐ Frequent dieting

☐ Anxiety associated with specific foods or meal skipping

☐ Chronic weight fluctuations

☐ Rigid rituals and routines surrounding food and exercise

☐ Feelings of guilt and shame associated with eating

☐ Preoccupation with food, weight, and body image that negatively impacts quality of life

☐ A feeling of loss of control around food, including compulsive eating habits

☐ Using exercise, food restriction, fasting, or purging to 'make up for bad foods' consumed

☐ Not being in tune with hunger or fullness cues or ignoring internal regulation cues in favour of external cues

☐ Food choices are strongly influenced by the desire to maintain a certain body size or shape

☐ Often eating to regulate emotions

☐ All-or-nothing approach with food

How many of these resonate with you? How many people in your life show signs of these, to some degree or another? Disordered eating is widespread – it doesn't just affect people who have eating disorders. Recognizing this is an important part of understanding the damage that diet culture has done to our relationship with food so that we can move towards something better.

What Is Intuitive Eating?

Intuitive eating is an evidence-based approach to food and eating developed in 1995 by Evelyn Tribole and Elyse Resch, two dieticians who were completely disheartened by using the traditional weight-loss model with their clients. Studies show that 80 per cent of weight is often regained within five years after being lost through a diet (see Chapter 1), so intuitive eating and a non-diet approach are focused on rejecting all forms of diet culture, as it often harms us more than it helps us.[5] Evelyn and Elyse define intuitive eating as a

> dynamic mind-body integration of instinct, emotion, and rational thought. It is a self-care eating framework – a personal process of honouring your physical and emotional needs by paying attention to the messages of your body. It is an inner journey of discovery that puts you front and centre; you are the expert of your own body. After all, only you know your thoughts, feelings and experiences. Only you know how hungry you are and what food or meal will satisfy you. No diet plan or guru could possibly know these things.

The intuitive eating model comprises ten principles:

1. Reject the diet mentality
2. Honour your hunger
3. Make peace with food
4. Challenge the food police
5. Feel your fullness
6. Discover the satisfaction factor
7. Cope with your emotions with kindness

8. Respect your body

9. Movement – feel the difference

10. Honour your health with gentle nutrition

Intuitive eating is a non-diet approach to health and well-being that helps you tune into your body's signals, break the cycle of chronic dieting (if it is present), and heal your relationship with food. It focuses on food freedom rather than food fear and is a powerful tool that helps to achieve health and well-being without the obsession. This approach gives you your power back over food. It empowers you to know that you, and you alone, have control over your own body and what makes you feel at your best. It focuses on internal, rather than external cues. It reconnects you with yourself and your needs. In short, it helps you unlock your inner wisdom. On a basic level, intuitive eating helps you to reprogram your relationship with food.

A non-diet approach takes the focus off weight loss and instead focuses on promoting health-enhancing behaviours, better body image, and a healthier relationship with food. To help guide eating choices, intuitive eating helps you get back in touch with internal cues, like hunger, fullness, and satisfaction. It also helps chip away at diet rules, like what, when, and how much to eat, so that you're better able to respond to your internal cues. A guideline that comes from inside the body is an internal cue, whereas one from outside the body is an external cue.

Intuitive eating helps to improve your interoceptive awareness or to remove barriers to your interoceptive awareness.

In other words, it helps you to cultivate attunement to physical sensations that arise from within your body in order to get both your biological and psychological needs met, or it removes the obstacles and disruptors to attunement, which usually come from the mind in the form of rules, beliefs, and thoughts. Interoceptive awareness is the ability to listen to physical signals from inside the body in the present moment and thus be able to respond to them.

For example, a physical cue could be hunger; a response to this is eating something. Another one could be feeling cold; a response would be to put on a jacket. Without being able to listen to these bodily cues, you will struggle to determine your needs and the correct response to those needs. Unfortunately, because of diet culture and many other reasons, it's really common to be completely disconnected from these signals, which is why my private practice (and this book) focuses on helping you reconnect with your body and these important cues. We're all born intuitive eaters, so even if you can't remember a time when you were connected to these cues, you definitely were. You just need to rediscover it.

How Is This Book Different?

This book draws heavily on intuitive eating, and I am indebted to Evelyn and Elyse for their trailblazing work. They are incredibly inspiring, and I've trained with them both — without them, I couldn't do what I do today. But this book is not based solely on the ten intuitive eating principles. I will leave that to the original book. This book is the result of the journey I have gone on, personally and professionally, to help my clients live a life of health and happiness without micro-managing their diet and lifestyle. Each chapter is inspired by the real-life obstacles that I see arise in my practice on a daily basis. The strategies I discuss have been used and validated by people struggling with the very problem you are facing right now. I help people just like you to leave dieting behind and rebuild their relationship with food, movement, and body image.

My professional qualifications range from nutritional science to intuitive eating, yoga, meditation, and psychotherapy. These qualifications have inspired the creation of this book, and they all get a look in. I have blended different elements of my expertise to develop the Remove, Reconnect, Re-establish system that aims to bring you from feeling stressed and obsessed about food to feeling calm and at ease and teach you how to begin improving your health when you get there. Many of my clients have told me that they feel a little lost as to how they can look after their health without dieting once they have done the work of healing their relationship with food; this book will show you how to do that through practical guidance. The Remove, Reconnect, Re-establish system has been years in the making, and I'm thrilled to share it with you in this book.

How This Book Works

This is important. Please don't skip this part.

There are three parts to this book that will help you reach your goal of feeling free from food and body image struggles. The system described here has arisen from my studies and experience as a food and body image counsellor and is informed by nutritional science, intuitive eating, mindfulness, psychology, and psychotherapy principles. Everything you read in this book is backed up by evidence and tested in real life on the thousands of people I have had the privilege of working with in my private practice through one-to-one relationships, group programmes, and workshops.

You may open this book, read the contents, and have the urge to skip to Part 3. Please don't do this. The first and second parts are imperative to approaching Part 3 with the mindset required to act on the recommendations in a sustainable way. Without first working through parts one and two of the book, the guidance given in part three will likely be taken on board like any other recommendations you've received from diet culture: like a set of rules and regulations. This book is different. This system is different. It's not about giving you more external rules to follow. Instead, it aims to put you back in control of food, and to be able to do that you will need to unlearn what holds you back and relearn what helps you flourish.

You might be thinking, 'Just tell me what to do, and I'll do it.' Firstly, has being told exactly what to do ever worked for you in the long term before? I wish rebuilding your relationship with food and body image was as simple as that, but unfortunately, it's not. That's why I've written this book — to give you a system to follow to help you get there. Here it is:

☐ **Part 1: Remove** — Remove what you've learnt from diet culture that keeps you stuck in a place of food stress and obsession and hinders your health and growth as a human being.

☐ **Part 2: Reconnect** — Reconnect with the needs of your mind and body to give you the information that you need to begin nourishing yourself with ease.

☐ **Part 3: Re-establish** — Re-establish health-promoting behaviours from this new perspective you've developed by first removing anything that does not serve you and then reconnecting with the needs of your mind and body.

The chapters have been laid out in this way for a reason, so I encourage you to read the book in sequence to get the most benefit. At the end of each chapter, I have added some comforting affirmations to support you with each step that you take towards food freedom. These affirmations correspond to the chapter at hand. Affirmations are a powerful tool that you can use to send positive messages to the subconscious parts of your brain, and doing so will help you to create a new mindset and belief system. Rejecting diet culture and rebuilding your relationship with food can be difficult. You are changing behaviours that may have been present for a lifetime. You are deconstructing an old belief system and creating a new one. Having some affirmations to hand when you come up against a challenging situation can be extremely helpful, so write them down or have them, somewhere close by so you can draw on them during these difficult moments. Then repeat them five times, either aloud or in your own mind.

At the end of the book is a section called 'Things to Remember'. Here you can record your key takeaways from the book, either chapter by chapter as you move through them, or at the very end. I recommend you do this as you go, since we tend to forget things quite quickly if we do not reflect on information within a few days.

A Few Things to Keep in Mind

Be compassionate with yourself
While navigating this process, you may begin unearthing things you did not expect. It's always about so much more than food. The reason why our relationship with food is so messed up in the first place is deeply rooted in oppression and patriarchy. This process can open your eyes to situations from your past and present that you begin to question, which can throw up emotions such as anger, shame, sadness, and guilt. Allow yourself to feel all of them. This is normal. There may also be moments where you struggle or hit bumps along the road. Embrace a mindset of curiosity and compassion when this happens. Please know that it is OK to feel uncomfortable along the way. Discomfort means growth. Remember that.

Let go of the timeline
There is no rush to have everything figured out by the time you finish this book. That's unrealistic. Healing is not linear; everyone moves at a different pace through this process. Let go of the idea that your relationship with food needs to be 'fixed' in a specific time period. That will only pressurize you and leave you open to disappointment.

Keep a journal
As mentioned above, I highly recommend you reflect on the

topics discussed in each chapter as you go. The 'Things to Remember' section provides some journalling questions you may wish to ask yourself as you move through the book. I cannot stress enough how beneficial journalling can be throughout this journey. Within the 'Things to Remember' section, there is space to write down your takeaways from each chapter, but it would be helpful to have a separate journal to expand on those take-aways and explore any other insights that arise as you move through the book. Your journal does not need to be fancy — it can be in digital form or hard copy, a fancy leather-bound book or a spiral notepad from your local shop.

Record your surprise wins
This is something you can do in your journal. Whenever you experience a win or something different to how you usually think about or behave around food — write it down. No win is too small — remember this. I like to call these 'surprise wins' because they often crop up at the most unexpected times. Then, if and when things get challenging, you can open up your journal and remind yourself how far you've come and why you're doing this.

Pause the pursuit of weight loss
If it feels manageable, I encourage you to pause any weight-loss efforts while you go through this process of rebuilding your relationship with food. If that feels uncomfortable for you, I get it, and I empathize with how difficult it can be to not actively pursue weight loss, especially if you live in a larger body. For my clients who feel this way, it helps them when I suggest putting a time frame on pausing the pursuit of inten-tional weight loss. Most people work with me for a minimum

of six months, so that often becomes their time frame. You can always go back to the pursuit of weight loss afterwards if you wish. For some people, the pursuit of weight loss may come with protection from stigma or oppression, and if this is the case for you, too, and you feel stuck, I highly recommend reaching out to a non-diet professional for support to help you make a decision that feels best for you.

Download the extra book resources
As you move through the book, you will be directed to a number of extra resources I have developed to help you on your journey to food freedom. These will be instrumental in helping you practically implement the content discussed. Head to nutritionwithniamh.com to download these and have them to hand as you move through each chapter.

Find a buddy or start a No Apologies *book club*
You may have one or more friends who would also like to rebuild their relationship with food. If so, set up some time to discuss your learnings or organize a book club to move through the book and process it together. Having peer support can be incredibly helpful if it's available to you. If not, don't worry – you can come and join my Facebook group to gain access to others on this journey. You'll find a link to this group in the book resources at nutritionwithniamh.com.

The Path to Food Freedom

Many people come to intuitive eating expecting that, once they have decided to stop dieting, they can move straight to becoming an intuitive eater. Unfortunately, that's not how it works. You cannot jump directly from dieting to eating intuitively. That's because intuitive eating is not another diet — it's the complete opposite. You must first heal from dieting, and only then will you be free to rediscover your intuitive eater. In order to create health and well-being, you must make space for a new story to emerge.

This process looks different for everyone. Every person that sits in front of me in clinic goes through a different process because they are all different people with a different life and set of past experiences. The more complex the history, the more complex the healing. One thing that's certain though, for everyone, is that rediscovering your intuitive eater and rebuilding a healthy relationship with food is the polar opposite of dieting. Dieting is easy at the beginning but gets harder and more unsustainable as time goes on. Intuitive eating can be difficult initially but gets easier and more sustainable as time passes.

I often compare dieting to hiking Everest. Taking those first few steps on the journey is the easiest part — it gets more difficult the further you trek and the higher you climb. All of the glory is at the top, when you summit the mountain. Since there are such low oxygen levels at the top, you can't stay there for long and must make the dangerous journey back down. This is much like dieting: you might be miserable the whole time, but the thrill of reaching your goal weight pushes you on. When you get there, however, it can feel very anti-climactic, especially when the weight you had worked so hard to lose begins to come back on. Eventually, you find yourself back at the place you started at — or worse, with more weight than you started with and an unhealthy relationship with food and body image to boot.

In contrast, intuitive eating is very much like a yellow brick road. Rather than all of the glory, winnings, and treasure being found at the end of the road, little pots of gold are found at every turn. These pots of gold then add up to a sizeable reward. Every obstacle or fork in the road is an opportunity for growth and learning. There are no mistakes, only learning experiences. Approach any obstacle or perceived failure with curiosity instead of judgement and ask yourself, 'What can I learn from this experience?' Doing so will teach you something about yourself and your relationship with food, even when you don't feel happy about the outcome. This is normal and all part of the process. Let's begin the journey.

PART 1: REMOVE

Remove what you've learnt from diet culture that keeps you stuck in a place of food stress and obsession and hinders your health and growth as a human being.

Chapter 1:

Deconstructing Diet Culture

When a past client of mine first came to work with me, one of the initial conversations we had, as is the case with most of my clients, was about deconstructing diet culture and the ways in which it shows up in our lives. She felt she had reached a stage of having rejected diet culture. She had begun to allow all foods in and live her life removed from the rules and regulations that had dictated her food choices for so long. Sure, she had some things she wanted to work on (which is why she had reached out to me for support), but she felt she had taken that critical and courageous first step towards food freedom. And she had. However, diet culture is a sneaky and slippery thing. It shows up in many ways, other than in guidelines of 'eat this' or 'don't eat that'. As with any slippery thing, just as we feel like we've got a hold of it, it can slither from our grasp once more. The question I always pose to my clients and continue to ask myself is 'Why?' Why do we feel a need to control our food intake, and where does it come from?

And what continues to feed the societal desire to be as slim as possible, often at a high cost?

This was the question that piqued my interest many years ago. It never sat quite right with me as a nutritionist to tell people what, when and how to eat. I deeply believe that there has to be an easier way to look after your health. I battled with this question at the beginning of my career. I felt a resistance to judging people's health based on their weight or advocating for reducing their lives to the pursuit of thinness if they were deemed 'overweight'.

Nevertheless, that's how I started my career. It was, in part, what I believed my job as a nutritionist would require. The weight-centric model of health has many strategies that attempt to eradicate fatness and unveil thinness, however unsuccessful these strategies may be. This was supported by societal beliefs and the conditioning I had been exposed to from an early age, as I'm sure you were too. When I began to question and challenge this belief system, I didn't like what I found and resisted it for some time before fully embracing it.

Nobody wants their deep-seated belief systems to be challenged. After all, I had started my nutrition training at the ripe age of 17, excited about the prospect of making a difference by helping our society fight the 'obesity epidemic'. I was born with thin privilege, which undoubtedly contributed to the opportunities that afforded me this possibility. Thin privilege represents the social, economic, political and practical advantages a person receives because they are thin or live in a relatively small body. My friend and yoga teacher Lucy Bloom often says, 'To invite in the new, we must let go of the old.' That's how it is with challenging belief systems, and growth is not always pretty. So I invite you to stay open, curious, and non-judgemental as you read on. The words and concepts within may challenge what you believe to be true. It may be utterly different from what you have considered true throughout your life, as it was for me. Stay with me and embrace the possibility of inviting in the new and letting go of the old.

What Is Diet Culture?

In the words of US dietician Christy Harrison, diet culture is 'a system of beliefs that equates thinness, muscularity, and particular body shapes with health and moral virtue; promotes weight loss and body reshaping as a means of attaining higher status; demonizes certain foods and food groups while elevating others, and oppresses people who don't match its supposed picture of "health".'[1] That's a lot more than the guidelines of 'eat this' and 'don't eat that', right? In its most basic form, it projects onto us the belief that 'thin is good' and 'fat is bad'. Diet culture upholds the beauty ideal and teaches us that we must look a certain way to be accepted and belong. Belonging is a basic human need. As social animals, we need to belong. This need may be unconscious, and many of us are unaware of it, but it resides within us all. Human beings are a tribal species, and to not belong means to die. In times gone by, when a community member was banished alone into the wild, they often didn't last long without their tribe. Although the development of civilization means that death by banishment is no longer a possibility, the need to be accepted and belong still rings true today. Diet culture feeds off our vulnerabilities and insecurities. We all experience a varying degree of expression of these vulnerabilities, due to the socio-cultural messages we have received both implicitly and explicitly about what it means to have a good body. The more insecure and vulnerable we are around food or our bodies, the stronger diet culture becomes.

Diet culture doesn't just sell you a diet. It sells you the elusive promise of health, happiness, success, desirability, and belonging. The result of dieting, however, is often far from that. Diet culture keeps you small and distracted by having you believe that your life cannot truly begin until you lose weight. This manifests in thoughts like 'I'll start dating when I'm thin,' 'I'll travel the world when I lose weight,' or 'I'll have a great social life/sex life/professional life when I drop x amount of dress sizes.' Unseen forces that contribute to these thoughts are also at play, such as societal oppression, which will affect how you see yourself and your body.

You alone cannot change society and rid yourself of these unseen forces, but we as individuals make up a collective. How you see yourself matters and contributes to collective change. A client I had been working one-on-one with for a few months told me that now she is more accepting of herself and others and no longer sees people as just fat, thin, and so on. The work she has done on rejecting diet culture will not just help her individually but will flow out of her in the way she thinks, feels, and behaves and will touch every person she meets. That's powerful stuff. What would the world be like if more of us thought in this way about ourselves and others? If we challenged diet culture and, as a result, became more compassionate people? What a fantastic world that would be! Change is possible, and it starts with you as an individual.

You cannot truly embrace food freedom and accept yourself as you are without understanding the perils of diet culture and learning how to reject it. Without doing this, there will always be a chain connected to a piece of you, threatening to pull you back down into the deep. This is why 'reject the diet mentality' is the first principle of intuitive eating. It's understandable to want to skip over the sticky bits of uncovering and challenging diet culture and the ingrained, often unconscious belief systems that many of us hold because of it. It can be uncomfortable and confronting. However, skipping this won't serve you, and it will most likely catch up with you down the road and sabotage your journey to food freedom. That's not to say that rejecting the diet mentality is a tick-box exercise that you complete in its entirety and move on. It's an ongoing process, since you will be faced with different forms of diet culture on a daily basis just by existing in the world as it is today.

The Roots of Diet Culture

To say no to diet culture, we must first understand its roots. When I began to challenge the deep-seated belief system of 'thin is good' and 'fat is bad', I was hungry to understand where our preference for thinness truly comes from. Would it surprise you to learn that our obsession with thinness only erupted in the nineteenth century? Although we can see some traces of fatphobia – a fear of fatness – in Ancient Greece and Rome, fat bodies were deemed beautiful, healthy, and desirable for much of history. In this period, the Latin word *obesus*, the root of the English word *obesity*, was coined, which translates to 'having eaten until fat'.[2] Between 1400 and 1700, the idea of female beauty was fat and full, exemplified in that era's popular art. In the nineteenth century, a shift occurred, and we started to see a trend of restricting women's body size. We began to see a mass standardizing of female beauty in Western culture and the promotion of unrealistic, unnatural body ideals. The corset, which was compulsory for aristocratic women in the sixteenth century, had by the nineteenth century become a hallmark of fashion for women of nearly all classes. The idealized hourglass figure that corsets provided was not possible without special garments, requiring women to work at making their bodies conform to unnatural measurements, despite the well-reported medical dangers of such.[3] As we can see, the trend of 'beauty at any cost' is not a new phenomenon.

Despite these developments, the voluptuous woman was still somewhat revered toward the end of the nineteenth century. Actresses such as Lillian Russell, who would fall into the 'obese' category of the body mass index (BMI) by today's standards, were widely admired.[4] However, the 'Gibson Girl', a new ideal who was slender in the waist and legs but still curvy in the hips and chest area, arose at the end of the nineteenth century and into the early twentieth century. From here on in, advertising and fashion continued to project an increasingly thin female beauty ideal that we still see enforced today, over a hundred years later.[5]

Diet culture as we know it today is rooted in racism, classism, and sexism. This may seem like a stretch to you, as it initially did to me, but it makes more sense once you begin to explore how fatphobia has developed over time. In her book *Fearing the Black Body*, Sabrina Strings writes about the racial origins of fatphobia and how the body began to be used to validate race, class, and gender prejudices. She writes of how

> two critical historical developments contributed to a fetish for svelteness and a phobia about fatness: the rise of the transatlantic slave trade and the spread of Protestantism. Racial scientific rhetoric about slavery linked fatness to 'greedy' Africans, and religious discourse suggested that overeating was ungodly . . . In the United States, fatness became stigmatized as both black and sinful. And by the early twentieth century, slenderness was increasingly promoted in the popular media as the correct embodiment for white Anglo-Saxon Protestant women.[6]

It was only after these associations were made that the effort to combat fatness developed into a major public health initiative. Strings goes on to explain how 'the phobia about fatness and the preference for thinness has not, principally or historically, been about health. Instead, they have been one way the body has been used to craft and legitimate race, sex, and class hierarchies.' The desire for thinness and fear of fatness is rooted in socio-cultural issues that are still prevalent today — albeit in somewhat less explicit ways. People who live in fat bodies are faced with macro- and microaggressions born out of weight stigma, just for simply existing. Weight stigma, the discrimination and oppression of fat people, originates from diet culture, which, as we have seen, ties body size to morality and goodness. Neither you nor I were born with the ideology that thinness makes you a better person. As we grew up, we learnt there are meanings attached to body size. We can see this in children – they will describe the people around them in an unfiltered way since they haven't yet learnt these meanings.

The roots of diet culture are also grounded in sexism. Despite men's increased preoccupation with thinness and muscularity and eating-disorder diagnoses, an imbalance leans further towards women, who face more significant pressure than men to look a certain way. In her book *The Religion of Thinness*, Michelle Lelwica outlines how gender roles have dictated body standards for men and women. She argues that men are encouraged to develop their minds, whereas women are taught to rely on their appearance. Men can pursue their dreams, while women must sacrifice their needs and desires for those around them.[7] These double standards are one of the reasons why more women are drawn into diet culture than men.

By understanding that fatphobia is a learnt behaviour rooted in centuries' worth of oppression and the creation of social and gender hierarchies so that some can prosper more than others, the prospect of removing diet culture as a driver of your thoughts and behaviours will become a more feasible endeavour.

What Is a Diet?

If diet culture is the system of beliefs that uphold beauty ideals, diets are the tools born of this system that it proposes should be used to eradicate fatness. A diet is anything based on a set of external rules that restricts what, when, or how much you eat in the pursuit of weight loss, 'wellness', or 'health'. It does not include autonomous choices you might make about food or those based on internal signals from within the body. For example, someone may choose to not eat meat because of their ethics or values. Another person may be bound to food restrictions for a medical condition, such as coeliac disease or allergies. Personally, I like to eat as much fruit and vegetables, whole grains and oily fish as possible because they make my body feel good. This is a choice that comes from a place of self-care rather than self-control. It is a choice that comes from within rather than a set of rules or regulations from the external world. Sure, it's supported by the benefits that I know these foods provide the body, but this is by no means the only reason I choose to eat them.

In contrast, dieting is all about control. It involves a creed or plan that must be followed to the letter. Anything less than this is deemed a failure. When we inevitably 'fall off the wagon', we blame ourselves, often beating ourselves with a large stick in the process. It's not uncommon for me to come across people in my clinic who feel like they're no longer dieting. This may be the case for some. However, dieting behaviours are so prevalent in our society that they can masquerade as normal eating. They're so widespread that it seems normal – but that doesn't mean it is. Dieting can constitute formal weight-loss diets, but it can also be informal, a compilation of all those rules, ideas and beliefs about food that you've picked up along the way. These rules intercept your connection to your intuition and can lead to you feeling lost around food.

For example, a client of mine had never actually been on an official diet. Still, she had received a lot of recommendations from gyms, personal trainers, and social media in the past that had constructed her beliefs around food. In her late teens, she loved banana and nut butter on toast in the morning. This is an excellent breakfast from a nutritional perspective, since it has a perfect balance of macronutrients, and most importantly, she enjoyed it; it satisfied her. A personal trainer she was working with told her that a banana wasn't the right choice as it had too much sugar. This is nonsense, but the seed was planted, and since then, she looked at bananas in fear and rarely ate them. And when she did, she felt guilty. This kind of problematic information is everywhere — it's next to impossible not to get caught out by it at some point, so please don't judge yourself if you have. Even if you've never formally dieted, you may have absorbed some of these messages too.

You may have noticed that dieting has fallen out of vogue over the last few years — we could even say that 'diet' has become a dirty word. Surely everyone knows by now that diets don't work? Maybe so, but diets are now operating under the guise of health and wellness, so they can be harder to spot. They've been dressed up in a way that seems to support health, but underneath, the premise is the same — a wolf dressed in sheep's clothing. I see this a lot on social media. 'It's not a diet; it's a lifestyle' springs to mind. Dieting has shape-shifted over the years and now shows up in the form of clean eating, plant-based, sugar-free, dairy-free — the list goes on. Christy Harrison calls this 'a diet by another name' in her book *Anti-Diet*. The wellness diet is all about eating the 'right' things and removing the 'wrong' ones, all in the name of correctness or health, which, of course, includes thinness and, as defined by Christy Harrison, 'is bound up in healthism: the belief that health is a moral obligation, and that people who are "healthy" deserve more respect and resources than people who are "unhealthy"'.[8] Be mindful of anything that is very rigid or puts boxes around what you should and shouldn't eat. Apply a critical lens to the information you receive around food and ask yourself why this proposed way of eating is better. If you struggle to answer that question or connect it to an internal cue, there is a good chance it's dieting in disguise. Here are few ways you can spot sneaky diet culture:

☐ Thinness is held up as an indicator of virtue

☐ Certain body types (e.g. 'the hourglass figure') are viewed as status symbols

☐ Weight is condemned as the direct cause of certain health conditions

☐ Foods are divided into 'good' and 'bad' categories

☐ Suggests cutting out certain types of food without a legitimate diagnosis

☐ Supportive of detoxes and/or cleanses.

If we dig into the 'why' behind these ways of eating, it's often grounded in the same weight-loss rhetoric and keeps us bound to eating by a set of rules and regulations. Here are some characteristics of dieters vs intuitive eaters to help you identify if your eating behaviours have been affected by dieting and diet culture:

Characteristics of Dieters	Characteristics of Intuitive Eaters
Rigid	Flexible
Eating is based on external cues	Eating is based on internal cues
Weight fluctuation	Stable weight
Disconnected from internal cues	Connected to internal cues
Compulsive overeating/ bingeing	Stops eating when satisfied
Feelings of guilt/shame	All foods permitted without guilt
Negative body image	Positive body image

The Diet Cycle

So what happens when you go on a diet? Let's walk through it together.

1. You hear about a new diet from someone who said it worked wonders for them. You say to yourself 'This one will be different' and get excited about the promised results. I get it.

2. The rules come next. You hit the gym, ditch the

carbs, and cut out all the 'crap'. You go all in on this new diet. You're doing so well. The weight starts to fall off and you feel amazing.

3. The water weight is gone and your weight loss starts to slow down. You become hypervigilant about labels, macros, calories, and so on. Perhaps you start to restrict yourself a little more to keep up the game.

4. Life happens and you just can't keep up with the exercise. The cravings start to take over and you say screw it and find yourself at the bottom of a tub of Ben & Jerry's.

5. You feel sick, guilty, and disgusted with yourself that you haven't been able to stick with the diet, yet again.

6. You might gain back some weight that you'd lost. So you're back at the start until you hear about the next new kid on the block and the restrict/binge cycle continues.

You don't fail the diet: the diet fails you. Diets don't work. Period. Dieting in order to fit a certain society-driven shape is a relatively new phenomenon, given the length of human existence. We are not all made from the same cookie cutter, nor should we be. Each person has a set-point weight that their body is happiest at, and trying to bring your weight too far below this will cause your body to constantly fight your efforts. When we eat for emotional reasons or don't pay attention to our inner intuitive signals, or if we experience a lifestyle change that contributes to weight gain, we may not be at our set point weight, or the weight at which our body is happiest and healthiest. Intuitive eating ditches the diets, heals the body from diet mentality, and helps your weight to stabilise at the place it's meant to be.

When our eating and the choices we make about food are wrapped up in food rules, restriction, deprivation, and good and bad foods, it feels the exact opposite of living a happy, fulfilling life. There is no such thing as a perfect way to eat, contrary to what Instagram and supposed gurus lead us to believe. Eating should not come with rules. It helps us to fuel and nourish our bodies and souls, forge connections with others, and, as Marie Kondo says, 'sparks joy'.

Dieting is bad for our physical, mental and emotional health, and there's a lot of scientific evidence to back that up. It's clear when we look at the science that there are more risks associated with dieting than benefits. Not only does dieting not work, i.e. it doesn't lead to long-term weight loss, but it also has some pretty undesirable side effects that intensify with every new diet embarked upon. Recognising that dieting *is* the problem will help to buffer against the widespread rhetoric that it's part of the solution.

Decreased metabolism
The body cannot tell the difference between dieting and actual starvation — it doesn't know when dieting is intentional or when there is a true food shortage that could threaten your survival. It compensates for the shortage of calories by lowering the body's need for energy. It does this by slowing

the metabolism, burning muscle for energy, and becoming uber-efficient at doing more for less. The body begins to store more fat in anticipation of the next diet, aka food shortage. One study showed that this effect on the metabolism could persist for six years after a diet![9]

Overeating and bingeing
Dieting leads to bingeing and overeating. When calorie intake is restricted, the brain sends out neurotransmitters and hormones like ghrelin and neuropeptide Y – powerful orexigenics that stimulate appetite. The production of these continue to rise until you eat enough to 'trip the switch' for the fullness hormone, leptin, to be released. Cravings will intensify. Basically, the body takes over and does everything it can to make you eat.

Loss of connection to internal cues
Dieters will more often rely on a self-imposed limit to stop eating, rather than relying on fullness cues. They will rely on a plan to tell them when to eat, rather than relying on internal hunger cues. They will choose food that is permitted, rather than tuning into satisfaction cues. When we rely on external cues to tell us when, what, and how much to eat, we lose trust in our own bodies to tell us what we need. We begin to rely on external rules and regulations to 'keep us on track'.

Increased food preoccupation
Most of the people that I work with say that food and body image take up 50–100 per cent of their daily head space. All you need to do is look and listen to the conversations

around you to collect evidence of this. We can see scientific evidence of this as far back as the Minnesota Starvation study, carried out in the 1950s, where college-age men who had no previous history of food or body image issues were put on a semi-starvation diet. Consequently, they spoke obsessively about food, with one man naming it 'nutritional masturbation'.[10]

Negative effects on self-esteem
Dieting chips away at your self-esteem, bit by bit. In 1992, at the National Institute of Health's Weight Loss and Control conference, psychological experts reported that dieting causes stress or makes the dieter more vulnerable to its effects. They also reported that it correlated with feelings of failure, lowered self-esteem, and social anxiety, independent of body weight itself. Dieting gradually erodes confidence and self-trust.

Long-term weight gain
Dieting causes long-term weight gain. Sure, you might lose weight initially through dieting, but many people will regain that weight, plus a little bit more, with every diet. How many people do you know who have sustained weight loss over a long period of time, i.e. longer than five years? The relationship between dieting and gaining back more weight is so strong that the Australian National Health and Medical Research Council rated it level 'A'. To give some context, the body of evidence available suggesting that smoking causes lung cancer is also graded level 'A'.

Increased risk of weight cycling
The constant yo-yo dieting, or gaining and losing weight from dieting, is known as weight cycling. Weight cycling itself is an independent risk factor for cardiovascular disease, inflammation, high blood pressure, and insulin resistance. Despite this, it is seldom controlled for in many large studies that associate weight with health issues.[11]

Dieting and Yang Energy

In my yoga teacher training, I first learned about yang and yin energy and the imbalance of yang energy present in today's world. Yang energy is doing; yin energy is being. Yang energy can also be referred to as masculine energy and yin as feminine energy. Both of these energies are present in us all, no matter if you are male or female. I know what you might be thinking: masculine energy must belong to males and feminine energy must belong to females. I understand why this might be your initial reaction to these terms, but I invite you to leave these assumptions aside as you read through the rest of this section. These words are simply descriptors to understand human behaviour on a deeper level. We can use these words as a tool rather than an absolute truth. We see the imbalance between these two energies played out not just in the inequalities between men and women but also in our unconscious drives as a society. As a people, we prioritise doing over being and reward achievement, even if this comes with great sacrifice and personal cost. Take the successful CEO who thrives in their career but feels overworked and lacks time to spend with family or have a family of their own. Or the award-winning business owner who left employment to enjoy time freedom but instead works 24/7 to make their business and themselves a success in the eyes of our capitalist culture. These are both real-life examples of the imbalance between yang (masculine) and yin (feminine) energy.

The terms 'feminine' and 'masculine' originate from the work of the psychiatrist Carl Jung, who first coined the terms 'anima' and 'animus' to reference the unconscious divine masculine and divine feminine energies that we all possess, no matter our gender. No matter the term used, whether it be feminine and masculine or yin and yang, I like to think of them as two different types of energy that need to be nurtured in order to thrive, grow, and fulfil your greatest potential. Both are important for optimum health and well-being. To be a well-rounded human being, we need to integrate both of these energies.

So what does this have to do with diet culture and dieting? Actually, a lot. Let me explain the characteristics of yang and yin energy to make this association clearer.

Yang (masculine) energy is:

☐ Action-oriented

☐ Assertive

☐ Boundaried

☐ Disciplined

☐ Logical

Yin (feminine) energy is:

☐ Intuitive

☐ Nurturing

☐ Reflective

☐ Compassionate

☐ Flexible

☐ Understanding

☐ Feeling

☐ Allowing

I can only speak for myself, but I wouldn't like having only one group of these characteristics as part of my personality — not having both would lead to clear deficits in quality of life. If we look at the attributes of yang energy, it doesn't take long to see these personified in the diets of today. They call on discipline, logic, and rigidity and dismiss intuition, reflection, and flexibility. They encourage the dismissal of yin energy and the messages you receive from the body through rules such as 'drink water to delay your hunger', 'have cauliflower instead of rice', or 'don't eat after 7 p.m.' The domination of yang energy materializes in the form of dieting through the message of 'make your body smaller at any cost'. The integration of yang and yin works in real life in such ways as:

> The yin says, 'I'm hungry.'
> The yang prepares food.
>
> The yin says, 'I'm cold.'
> The yang grabs a blanket.
>
> The yin says, 'I'm feeling sad and lonely.'
> The yang calls a friend.
>
> The yin says, 'I need help.'
> The yang reaches out for support.

Being connected to both of these energies within yourself is crucial for getting your needs met. Having a direct line to your intuition, understanding the messages your body is giving you and allowing yourself to follow through with an action that reflects those needs are all critical parts of a healthy relationship with food and your body. Therefore, whether you are male or female, the journey towards rebuilding that relationship will involve getting back in touch with your yin energy, which may have been dismissed for quite some time. As I have seen with many of my clients, it may be lost, but it can be found again with some support and guidance, leading you to health, happiness, and alignment.

Exploring the Evidence

I've come on my own journey of rejecting diet culture and moving from weight-centric to weight-inclusive practice. I'm a scientist first and foremost, and it was drilled into me throughout my degree to always look for the evidence behind any recommendations or advice, and rightly so. Evidence-based practice is the holy grail in nutritional science and will continue to be an essential part of my professional practice. These ethics and values guided me when I began to delve into the science behind dieting — and wow, was I surprised. This inquiry cracked open all I had previously taken as truth and failed to question.

On the one hand, it threw up an existential crisis within my career, and on the other hand, it opened up a whole new world that I never knew existed. It opened up the possibility of helping people work on their health without being hyper-focused on weight. I hadn't worked very much in weight management up to that point, but the people I did work with from a weight-loss capacity initially lost weight through the plan I suggested but eventually gained it back. I carried out thousands of body composition checks with people over four years and sat with the shame they felt after being deemed 'overweight' or 'obese'. These were focused, dedicated individuals who excelled in other areas of life — why was this different? Was it all down to the individual, or was there more to the story? These early experiences in my career were a thread I couldn't help but pull on, and it all made sense when I began to look into the evidence. Moving away from dieting in a world that tells you that being thin is one of the most important things you can be is radical, so we need to build a case for why we should even do so in the first place. That's where exploring the evidence comes in.

Exploring the Science Behind Dieting

Now for the ugly truth: diets don't result in long-term weight loss. When I say long term I am referring to a time period of more than five years. For all the headlines you see touting the benefits of this diet over that diet and the ample before and after pictures you see on social media, there is not one single study available showing that permanent weight loss is possible for more than a small percentage of people. If you have experienced yo-yoing weight throughout your life, please know that it is not your fault, and there is more to this than 'willpower'. If I could choose just one message for you to leave this book with, it would be this: it's not your fault that all those diets you've tried in the past haven't worked.

There is a narrative supported in our society that to be 'overweight' or 'obese' is a character flaw and down to individual responsibility. Yes, there's no denying that your diet and lifestyle influence your weight, but the idea that it can be controlled entirely is outdated and not reflected in the research. Some people are born with thin privilege and will remain that way throughout their life. Others are not. We know that 50 to 70 per cent of body weight is genetically determined. That means that your weight is not solely determined by the decisions you make around diet and lifestyle. Up to 80 per cent of your height is genetically determined, yet it would seem ludicrous to try and change the height you've been given at birth.[12] Nevertheless, we are sold the elusive promise from diet culture that you can control your weight if you try hard enough (just buy this diet plan, right?). In reality, intentional weight-loss efforts don't work in the long term, with a failure rate of 95 to 98 per cent.[13] This statistic originates from one of the original studies that evaluated outpatient treatment for 'obesity' by Albert Stunkard in 1959. Of course, one small study does not make an evidence base, but since then, science has continued to back up these findings that diets do not result in long-term and sustained weight loss for most people:

☐ A 2015 study of more than 278,000 people found that within five years the proportion of people who've regained all their lost weight (or more) after a diet is between 95 and 98 per cent. The same study found a 0.004 per cent chance for men and a 0.01 percent chance for women of attaining a 'normal' BMI, between 20 and 25, for those with a BMI over 30. For those with a BMI between 40 and 45, the probability dropped to 0.0008 percent for men and 0.001 percent for women.[14]

☐ A 2007 meta-analysis of weight-loss studies found that people's weight usually reaches its lowest point somewhere around the six-month mark of any diet or 'lifestyle change'; it then starts increasing at about one year, after which the rate of weight regain speeds up over time.[15]

☐ A 2020 review of weight-loss studies with at least a three-year follow-up found that the average rate of weight regain is 0.14 per cent each month, meaning that the average participant will reach their starting weight within four years. This result is consistent with other studies showing that most people regain the weight they lost (if not more) in about five years.[16]

☐ A 2013 study analysed every single randomised controlled trial (the gold standard) of weight-loss interventions that included a follow-up of at least two years and found that dieters lose weight in the first year, only to gain back all but an average of 2.1 pounds over the next two to five years. Not only this, but just twenty-one studies met the criteria for a follow-up longer than two years — a very low number, given the assumption of many that almost anyone can lose weight and keep it off.[17]

All that blood, sweat and tears for a measly two pounds! I don't know anyone who would be happy with that outcome when embarking on a weight-loss diet — it's common for your weight to fluctuate around two pounds in a single day! I could continue to talk about the science for pages and pages, but I feel that this snapshot gets the message across: diets don't work.

Exploring Your Personal Experiences

Are you heavier, lighter, or the same weight since you started dieting? What has your personal experience with dieting been? To help my clients understand this more deeply, I often suggest they complete a diet history. This involves writing down all the diets you have done throughout your lifetime (as many as you can remember — there may be a lot) and being honest with yourself about whether or not each of these diets led to long-term weight loss. This part of exploring the evidence requires you to close the gap between fantasy and reality. If weight loss occurred, for how long was it maintained? Did you gain more weight than you lost after the diet ended? These are the kinds of questions to ask yourself that can help you build a case for change against dieting. Asking yourself these questions may bring up a lot of emotions. Anger and sadness are the most common ones I see when working through this with my clients. This is normal. Be compassionate with yourself as you explore your past experiences and know that you can channel these emotions and direct them towards developing a plan to change.

Exploring the Experiences of Others

A few years ago, I led a workshop with over a hundred women ranging from age 20 to 60. I asked them several questions about their experiences with dieting and the pursuit of intentional weight loss. Very quickly, it became clear that most of the room had similar experiences. These women were of different ages. They were at completely different stages of life. They each had their own story. Yet they all had the same experience when it came to dieting: in the long term, they had gained weight, not lost it. Their experiences mirrored the science.

Think about the people in your life. Do you know anyone who has lost weight and maintained that weight loss for more than five years? If the answer is yes, are these people in the majority or the minority? When I ask my clients this question, they often say they don't know anyone who has maintained substantial weight loss. One person in an intimate workshop I led on intuitive eating said she knew someone who had. When she shared this with me, I asked her if she had any insight into what her life was like. Silence. And then an answer came: 'Yeah, not great.' For many people who have maintained weight loss for more than five years, the work and sacrifices to do so are staggering. For most people, maintaining weight loss does not come without significant costs.

I know all of this might be hard to hear, and you may still feel sceptical or be in a state of denial reading this. I get it. On the other hand, if this is shocking you and you feel despondent, angry, and let down as a result, please don't lose hope. This rollercoaster of emotions is normal when you become aware of the facts. There are many things you can do to improve how you feel in your body, and practising health-promoting behaviours consistently will contribute to long-term health benefits, while allowing your weight to settle within a healthy and happy weight range that is right for your body.

Diet Culture Detection

When I speak to clients in my private practice about rejecting diet culture, I share how it needs to be first detected in both your internal and external world if you want to reject it successfully. A word of warning: once you see diet culture, you will see it everywhere. Acclaimed American author David Foster Wallace made a speech in 2005 containing the following anecdote:

There are these two young fish swimming along, and they happen to meet an older fish swimming the other way, who nods at them and says, 'Morning, boys. How's the water?' And the two young fish swim on for a bit, and then eventually, one of them looks over at the other and goes, 'What the hell is water?[18]

When they begin to detect diet culture, many of my clients are amazed at how they've never seen it before. Often the most prominent, ubiquitous, and important realities are the ones that are difficult to identify. Just as the fish did not realize they were swimming in the water, you may not have realized how ubiquitous diet culture truly is. Once this realization is reached, there truly is no turning back. We believe what we have been taught to believe. If we've been taught that something is true and correct, we rarely take the time to reflect and fact-check that piece of information. This is the case with many different belief systems and is clear to see when we look at cultural differences. Take the Spanish siesta, for example. The siesta is a short nap taken in the early afternoon, often after the midday meal. It's part of Spanish tradition. The first time I visited Spain, this shocked me because I believed that people didn't take naps in the middle of the day, right? Some people do; my culture had just taught me they didn't.

Without the ability to detect diet culture in your internal and external environment, you will be open and vulnerable to its messages. This step is all about armouring yourself against those messages and calling them out for what they are. Let's say you're heading out for the day. If you live in Ireland, you'll be checking the weather before you leave the house to see if rain has been forecast. If it has (or even if it hasn't because, hey – Irish weather!), you'll bring along an umbrella. Without the umbrella, every raindrop will be absorbed into your clothes if you get caught in a rain shower. Learning the skill of detecting diet culture is a little like having an umbrella to protect you from the rain. Instead of absorbing all of its messages, it will slide right off your umbrella, like water off a duck's back. Here are some questions you can ask yourself to help spot and call out diet culture:

☐ Is it shrouded in shoulds, musts and have-tos?

☐ Can you fail or break rules?

☐ Is it based on external cues or a meal plan? (with the exception of some medically recommended diets or within an eating disorder recovery plan)

☐ Do you have to count anything like points, macros, or calories?

☐ Are you being told what, when, and how much to eat?

☐ Are you being advised to cut a food or food group out without a medical diagnosis?

All of the above teach you that you cannot be trusted around food and need external rules to keep you 'on track'. They bring you further away from your hunger and fullness cues and instead create a preoccupation and reliance on psychological, cultural, or social signs to eat – which is why we want to detect its presence.

How to Reject Diet Mentality

You cannot reject the diet mentality if you do not first understand why you're doing so. Accepting that diets don't work in the long term is the first step toward rebuilding a healthy relationship with food and body image. Rejecting diet mentality will not happen overnight — it's a process you will build on over time.

Think about it like this. Inside your mind sits a queen on her throne, who has ruled the land of your mind for many years. She has an army of strong soldiers that support the messages of diet culture. Each time you reject the diet mentality through any of the steps outlined below, it's as though you take one of those soldiers into your new army of defectors. This queen will not want to give up her throne, so you will win some battles and lose others. Every time you claim one of her soldiers as a defector, please celebrate this as a victory, and when diet mentality wins some of the battles, remind yourself that you're playing the long game. Over time, the old army will get weaker, and the new army will get stronger. Trust that it will become easier to detect and reject diet mentality as time goes on. This is down to neuroplasticity, the ability of the brain to form new pathways and connections. In other words, the brain becomes rewired to function differently from how it has operated in the past. Every time you claim a soldier into your new army, you're creating a new pathway in the brain, and every one of those instances counts. We know that mindfulness contributes to neuroplasticity and changes the brain's physical structure and, therefore, changes the way we think, feel, and act, which is why it's our first step.

Step 1: Become aware of diet mentality thoughts
When it comes to detecting and rejecting diet culture internally, mindfulness is a key skill you will need to cultivate. In the words of Jon Kabat-Zinn, 'mindfulness is paying attention to something, in a particular way, on purpose, in the present moment, and non-judgementally'.[19] You can use mindfulness to create some mental space and gain an insight into the thoughts percolating in your mind. A human being has approximately 60,000 thoughts in a day! It goes without saying that you won't be able to catch them all as they pass through your mind, no matter how skilled a mindfulness practitioner you become. But you will become more proficient at noticing some thoughts and, as a result, aware of those that fall into the camp of diet mentality. The chances are that the same diet mentality thoughts will arise repeatedly.

My experiences with yoga were my entry point into mindfulness. When I first learnt you could become an observer of your thoughts, it was a real lightbulb moment for me. What I'd like you to do at this moment is close your eyes and say hello to yourself in your mind three times. Can you hear yourself saying it? Of course you can! Welcome to being mindful. Mindfulness can be formal, in the case of meditation, or informal, such as when you notice saying hello to yourself inside your mind. It may also involve bringing awareness into every day by becoming aware of your thoughts, feelings, and behaviours or stepping into the senses by noticing what you can see, hear, smell, touch, or taste. It is simply the act of conscious living.

I like to think of the mind as a glasshouse. Visualize yourself standing outside this glasshouse looking in. Inside this glasshouse, lots of butterflies are flying around. These butterflies represent your thoughts. Some of these butterflies will be easy to catch; others not so much. Becoming aware of and catching these butterflies is akin to mindfulness of thought, and the more you practise, the better you will become.

When you notice diet mentality thoughts, it may be helpful to give them a name or call them out as 'diet culture', a process called externalization. When thoughts are externalized, you separate them from yourself — they are not a part of you. Through this act of separation, it becomes easier to see where you end and diet culture begins. Diet mentality thoughts are usually shrouded in shoulds, musts, and have-tos. They could sound like:

'I really want the pizza, but I'm being good today.'

'I'm hungry, but it's 7 p.m., so I can't eat any more.'

'If I don't exercise, I'll gain weight.'

'This is healthy, and I should enjoy eating it as it will make me thin.'

'I can't trust myself around food, so I must restrict what and how much I eat.'

Step 2: Reframe diet mentality thoughts
Once you catch diet mentality thoughts, the next step is to reframe them without a side of diet culture. Reframing diet mentality thoughts will begin the process of neuroplasticity explained above. You can draw on many things to help you reframe sneaky diet culture thoughts. Here are some examples to guide you:

Using a realistic mindset

Diet mentality: 'I really want the pizza, but I'm being good today'.

Reframe: 'Obsessing about the pizza is unhealthy. It's just food. Eating pizza all the time wouldn't make my body feel well but allowing myself to have it is OK and part of a healthy relationship with food.'

Using your past experiences

Diet mentality: 'I can't trust myself around food, so I must restrict what and how much I eat.'

Reframe: 'Of course I feel out of control around some foods! I have been restricting them for years. While I have some evidence that overeating has happened in the past in response to giving myself freedom around food, the restriction is what caused it. More restriction is not the answer.'

Using your lived experience

Diet mentality: 'My friends are all on a new diet I haven't tried before. Mary has lost so much weight and looks amazing. Maybe I should give dieting one last go . . .'

Reframe: 'There will always be a new diet to tempt me. I've done so many diets in the past. They all end in the same outcome – long-term weight gain. Sure, I did lose some weight initially, but it eventually returned, and I was left preoccupied with food and my body anyway.'

Step 3: Ditch the diet tools
Diet tools can come in many forms; here are some examples:

- ☐ Calorie or fitness trackers (sometimes, these may be used for other means beside weight control)

- ☐ Weighing scales

- ☐ Diet books

- ☐ Clothes that haven't fit in over twelve months

- ☐ Diet-y social media accounts

- ☐ Weighing or measuring food before eating it

- ☐ Exercise as compensation for foods eaten

These externalize success and base motivation on extrinsic factors rather than intrinsic ones. I practise a person-centred counselling approach, so bodily autonomy is always top of my values list. When people question whether they should stop using any of the above, I always ask how these tools make them feel and what the short-term and long-term outcomes are of using them. If their use leads to stress, worry, or anxiety, they have no place in your journey back to food freedom. Allow the messages from within to guide you towards the correct answer for you.

Step 4: Challenge diet talk
Rejecting the diet mentality can make you feel like you're swimming against the tide in a world preoccupied with external appearance. Many people in your life may not be on the same journey as you towards a healthy and relaxed relationship

with food. Being faced with the opinions of others can be challenging and cause you to question your decision to move away from dieting. This is normal, and coming up against diet mentality in your external environment is expected, so you'll need some tools to tackle these instances. Calling out diet culture externally is the same as internally: 'this is diet culture'.

There are four main ways that you can deal with diet talk. I have learnt that it's not my responsibility to educate every person I come across about the perils of diet culture. I would burn out if I did this, so I'm very strict about my boundaries to protect my energy. Some people are more outspoken than others, and that's OK. You need to do what feels right for you at any given moment. One of my clients, who has successfully rejected diet culture, found it helpful to categorize the diet talk she was faced with, which helped her prepare for them when they arose. Here are some potential responses when faced with diet talk:

1. Ignore
Many of my clients will feel most comfortable ignoring diet talk at the start of their journey. You can do this by deciding not to participate in the conversation or leaving the room by excusing yourself to the bathroom. If it feels inappropriate to leave, move on to option two.

2. Change the subject
A conversation requires two or more people, so changing the subject will remove the fuel needed to keep the topic alight. Over time, other people will begin to understand that you are not someone who participates in diet talk, and they will get bored with starting these

conversations with you. You may have been someone that initiated these conversations in the past, and in this case, it will take time for this to happen.

3. Plant a seed

Share some of your new-found awareness of diet culture and the different mindset you are cultivating. This can be done by sharing some of your own experiences or making suggestions about where they could learn more about intuitive eating and diet culture – such as a podcast or this book! When my clients ask me how to explain this to friends or family members, I usually tell them to share my podcast, 'Food, Body and Beyond'. This takes the pressure off you while still getting your point across. It doesn't often turn out well when we accuse someone else of being wrong or act in a way that brings out their defences. To avoid this, you could say something like, 'I'm reading this great book/listening to this podcast/following this social media page that's changed my perspective on this topic if you're interested?'

4. Set a boundary

If steps one, two, and three continue to fail, it may be time to set a boundary, especially if the diet talk you face is frequent and triggering for you. We will talk more about boundaries in Part 3, but here are some examples to get you started:

Diet talk: You really shouldn't eat that – it's got so many calories!

Boundary: Please don't comment on what I do or do not eat.

Diet talk: You've lost so much weight/gained so much weight since I've seen you last!

Boundary: Those kinds of comments make me uncomfortable. I'd appreciate it if you didn't comment on my weight.

Diet talk: Let me tell you about this fantastic new diet I'm on . . .

Boundary: I really like catching up with you, but I'd rather not talk about weight and dieting. What else have you been up to recently?

At the start of this process of rejecting the diet mentality, it may feel like it's taking up a lot of bandwidth. When you learn any new skill, the beginning is slow, hard work, and then one day it becomes so easy you could do it your sleep. Keep at it, and I promise you'll get there.

Affirmations

Dieting causes me to gain weight, not lose weight.

I am working on rejecting diet culture.

I am compassionate towards myself throughout this process.

I am doing my best, and that is enough.

I release all feelings of regret.

I am worthy of love and respect, no matter my size.

Chapter 2:

Detaching from Appearance Ideals

Holidays are a time when many photo opportunities arise — in front of monuments, on the beach, while out for dinner, hiking a mountain: this is when the camera often comes out. If I have learnt one thing over the years working with people who struggle with body image (spoiler alert: most of the female population and a large percentage of the male population), it is that photos are a tricky subject. They can trigger a whole host of insecurities and inadequacies a person feels about their appearance, size, or body shape. I have definitely fallen victim to becoming consumed by thoughts over a particular photo and how I appear in it. Many clients have shared the same experience, not to mention the number of times I've witnessed friends and family agonizing over photos too. The phrases I often hear (and have said myself) are:

'Ugh, that's an awful photo.'

'Delete that!'

'I look huge!'

'I can't even recognize myself.'

'Do I really look like that?'

Have you ever questioned where these insecurities or perceived inadequacies come from? Do young children dwell on photographs in the same way we do as teenagers or adults? Do they poke at their dimples, belly rolls, or double chin? Of course they don't, because they have yet to learn that there is such a thing as 'good' and 'bad' bodies. Disliking your body is not something you are born with. It's something you have been taught to do. We are all born fully embodied and connected to our bodies. Watch any baby or toddler to gain an insight into the relationship you once had with your body.

We are a world obsessed with external appearance. The age of social media has only exacerbated that, and very few people are immune. This obsession leads us to resort to all sorts of measures to try and live up to these standards society has set for us — I could fill a book just with these measures alone. But of course, no matter how many measures you enlist, it's never enough. That's because we have been conditioned to look for flaws; god forbid if you accept the body you have today and live a fulfilling life regardless — sacrilege! No, you must always be trying to enhance, tone, slim, or change your body and, let's not forget, defy the ageing process.

As I write this, I can feel my heart beating and tears forming in my eyes for two reasons: I feel both sad and outraged that this is what we are subjected to. *This* is the core of why we have such a messed-up relationship with food in the first place.

Controlling your food intake has been sold as the golden ticket to fit into the thin ideal you've been taught you need to live up to so you can be deemed worthy and valued by society. I call bullshit. This is why I speak to so many people who feel inadequate and are under so much pressure to conform. Why there have been so many missed opportunities and sacrifices made. When focusing on your appearance comes at a high sacrifice or personal cost, it's time to ask questions.

The issue here is that, in our quest to attain the beauty ideal, we say no to things we truly desire and instead remain consumed and distracted by a journey with no destination. There is no destination because no amount of changes you make to your body will ever be enough. It's as if just before you reach the finish line, the finish line shifts, and there's a new one to aim for. We know that weight loss, for example, does not improve negative body image. Some people have lived their whole life this way – maybe you, reading this right now, have too. This is not your fault, and there is a way out.

Beauty and Appearance Ideals

I was fifteen when I had my first experience with dieting, a tender age for most young girls. I felt as though my body wasn't enough, and I would be happier when I was skinnier. I believed this with a vigorous intensity – nobody could have convinced me differently. I thought that any worries, fears, or insecurities would evaporate if I could just be smaller. Alas, even when I did become smaller, that never happened – shocker! Most people, especially women, have had a similar experience to mine in their life, some at a much younger age than others. I have worked with people who have memories of feeling this way from as early as age four.

Thankfully, I had a very healthy relationship with food growing up (thanks, Mam and Dad — they'll be delighted to get a mention here). I believe that this, along with my thin privilege, protected me in part from an escalation of those early experiences with dieting in my teens. The main reason for flirting with dieting in my teenage years was the exposure to unattainable appearance ideals in mainstream media. The next step in removing what you have learnt from diet culture is to honestly examine the appearance and beauty ideals that we've all been subjected to and the role that these unattainable ideals play in keeping you stuck chasing a specific body size or shape. Without challenging the status quo and working on respecting and accepting your here-and-now body, you will struggle to truly reject the diet mentality, find food freedom, and feel better about yourself as a person.

Firstly, what's wrong with chasing beauty ideals? Well, for one, it can be pretty damn miserable, but apart from that, they constantly change, so it's impossible to reach them. Our bodies are not lumps of clay we can sculpt and mould to any size or shape, despite what we've been led to believe. Prior to the 1900s, the beauty ideal for women in Western culture was voluptuous and soft — a larger body was seen as beautiful. This beauty ideal began to shift once we entered the twentieth century. Let me give you a whistle-stop tour of how female beauty ideals have shifted over the past hundred years or so.

1900s: Women of all classes began to wear corsets to emphasize curves and a small waist.

1920s: Curves are de-emphasized, and a skinny female body came into fashion.

1940s: The fuller hourglass figure, known as the 'pin-up', becomes popular.

1960s: Thin is in again.

1980s: Having a fit and 'toned' body is ideal. Slim, but also strong.

1990s: Thin, pale, young-looking and waif-like.

2020s: Thin but curves in the 'right places'. Big bum and breasts.

I'm exhausted just reading this. How are we supposed to keep up? We can't, and that's the point. Chasing beauty ideals keeps us distracted and suppressed because of the time and energy required to diet. We cannot buy any more time or energy; it is a finite resource. If the majority of it is given over to dieting, it has to be taken from somewhere else. Not to mention the money spent on diet products; many of my clients tell me they could buy a small car with the money they've spent dieting. When we spend our time trying to mould and shape ourselves into an acceptable physical form, we lose sight of the things that truly matter and lose time playing a game we can never win.

As you can see above, thinness in some form has dominated beauty ideals since the 1900s, but a thin body is not earned. You cannot will yourself thin. Of course your body shape and size is influenced by the food you eat and the lifestyle you maintain, but they're not the only things that have an impact, as we spoke about in Chapter 1. Life is short, and every day you spend trying to live up to an unattainable ideal is time wasted. This pursuit distracts you from focusing on things that make you truly happy, such as inner health and contentment, nurturing relationships, or a fulfilling career. The pursuit of the beauty ideal does not come without sacrifices. As you continue to opt out of diet culture, you might need to come back to this point again and again. What are you giving up to pursue thinness and are those sacrifices worth it to you? Only you can answer this question.

Self-Objectification Theory

When we are exposed to unattainable beauty ideals, which most of us are from a very young age, we learn to measure and compare ourselves to these. In other words, we begin to self-objectify. In their book *More Than a Body*, Lexie and Lindsay Kite describe how

> self-objectification occurs when people learn to view their own bodies from an outside perspective, which is a natural result of living in an environment where bodies are objectified. We grow up seeing idealized and sexualized female bodies presented in media as parts for others' viewing pleasure, even in the most mundane or unexpected circumstances. In 1975, film theorist Laura Mulvey coined the term 'the male gaze' to describe the phenomenon of women being represented in media through the perspective of a heterosexual man, in which they are sexualized and depicted as passive objects of male attention or

desire. This is objectification. We then learn to monitor and understand our own bodies from the same outside perspective. This is self-objectification. When we are self-objectifying, our identities are split in two: the one living her life and the one watching and judging her.[1]

This splitting of our identity leads us to become the seer and the seen – we live both within our bodies and judge ourselves from the outside. Lexie and Lindsay, two body image researchers, explain how our first experience of this arises when we wade into the sea of objectification. This can happen in a multitude of ways: hearing a family member disparage their own body; experiencing cat-calling on the street; watching Disney princess movies and noticing that none of the female characters look like you or anyone you know; receiving unsolicited comments from adults about your body, either positive or negative; or simply noticing which girls or boys got the most attention in your class at school. As a young child, before we are exposed to these experiences, we live on the more-than-a-body beach, where we exist unapologetically and in a carefree way. When you start to recognise the objectification of bodies, whether in the media or through personal experience, your perception of yourself becomes divided; there's the whole, embodied you, and the self-objectifying part of you.

I like to think of self-objectification as having an 'other' that is with you at all times. The only job of the 'other' is to compare the way that you look to the 'ideal body' and look out for the ways in which you don't measure up. The 'other' is like a little devil on your shoulder, whispering things in your ear like:

'You're not thin enough.'

'You're not tall enough.'

'You have wrinkles. You should fix that.'

'Ugh, cellulite.'

'Your muscles aren't big enough.'

'You're too old.'

Need I go on? You get the picture, right? I have no doubt you will identify with this concept and notice what your own internal self-objectifying voice of the 'other' sounds like. This voice is a result of all the messages you have internalized about what the ideal body should look like. We will shine a spotlight on this voice and you will learn how to begin tackling it in Chapter 4.

Hillary McBride, a psychologist, shares her 'moving onto the front lawn' analogy in her book *The Wisdom of Your Body* to further explain this process of self-objectification and how it interferes with embodiment. This metaphor is one that blew my mind when I first discovered it and is one that I have adapted for use with my clients in clinic.

Your body is your home; the only home you'll ever have. If you're one of the lucky ones, it comes equipped with everything you need to carry you through this life; lungs to breathe, a heart to pump blood around your body, muscles to walk and lift objects, a brain to think and disseminate information and a digestive system to receive and utilize energy. Now let's compare your body to a house. Inside your house, you have a fully stocked fridge, a bed to sleep on, a shower to clean yourself, and a cosy couch to relax in. Just like the way you viewed your body with amazement as a toddler, you view your house as having everything you could possibly need. That is until you learn to judge your body from the outside and that it should be continually fixed or enhanced. Until you begin to peer out the front window of your house and see all your neighbours out on their front lawn, judging their houses from the outside. As described by Hillary:

> You were content living life inside your house until the compelling dialogue about colours, shapes and house sizes drew you outside. Pretty soon, you start spending more time outside on the lawn comparing your house to the other houses. Your house doesn't look quite like it used to, so you start doing what you can to fix it up. When people notice the changes and comment, it feels good. Pretty soon, you find yourself spending more time on your front lawn than you do inside your house.[2]

Your house was designed for you to live inside of it, not outside. You can design or decorate your house whatever way you like, without apology, because it's your house and nobody else's. In fact, life would be very boring if everyone's house looked the same, right? Spending all of your time out on the front lawn only robs you of enjoying your house and using it as it was intended:

> When it comes to our bodies, most of us are living on the front lawn. We are looking at our bodies from the outside only, and we have not yet learned how to move back in.[2]

Look around; how many people do you know that have been conditioned to live in this way? Most people. But if we spend all our time outside on the front lawn, we can't know what is happening inside the house. We lose connection to our inner expert. We become disembodied. A large part of developing a positive body image and, as a result, moving closer toward food freedom is to examine and reject these messages that our value and worth lie in external appearance. This allows us to move back into the home that we were always destined to inhabit.

But What if I Want to Lose Weight?

Having a desire for weight loss is normal in our current culture. Most people who seek out intuitive eating have a desire to lose weight. After all, the universal focus on weight loss is one of the reasons why we become disconnected from our intuitive eater in the first place. People embarking on a journey of rebuilding their relationship with food and body image often ask me whether they need to rid themselves of this desire. It's not as simple as this, unfortunately; you cannot flick a switch and no longer have the desire to lose weight, especially if you have been told your whole life that this is something you must do to be healthy and happy. Therefore, it's perfectly acceptable to have this desire, but you can choose whether or not to act on it.

Relinquishing your desire for weight loss is not a prerequisite for embarking on this journey, but acting on that desire by actively pursuing weight loss through dieting is.

Depending on your mindset or life circumstances, this may or may not feel incomprehensible to you. Evelyn Tribole and

Elyse Resch, the founders of intuitive eating, explain how one needs to hit diet bottom before becoming available to embrace the process of fully rediscovering their intuitive eater. Hitting diet bottom occurs when you are painfully aware that every diet you have done up until that point has ended in 'failure', and any weight you previously lost has been regained (if not a little bit more with every diet). You may be consumed by thoughts and worries around food and body image and are tired of living a life dictated by the scales. Your self-worth may feel very attached to your weight and external appearance. This will continue until you decide you are tired of living this way – a way you may have been living for years or even decades. It may feel scary to move away from dieting, and deciding not to pursue weight loss in service of your long-term health and well-being can be difficult. However, it is necessary to truly heal and rebuild your relationship with food and body image. Pursuing weight loss while trying to rebuild your relationship with food is a little like trying to go to Dublin and Cork simultaneously – you can't.

I always say this tentatively because I know the gravity of what I am suggesting. Whether or not you face systemic oppression or weight stigma may also make this decision more challenging, but it is possible; I have seen people of all shapes and sizes reclaim their intuitive eater and achieve body acceptance. This doesn't mean weight loss is not discussed – it often is in my virtual clinic room. We need to create lots of non-judgemental space and compassion for this process, especially if it's something that has provided you safety and reprieve from oppression. If you are reading this and struggle with the idea of pausing your pursuit of weight loss, I highly suggest getting support from a non-diet and health at every size (HAES)-aligned nutritionist, dietician, or therapist. Healthcare professionals that have trained in this area and work in a weight-inclusive way will be able to help you move towards a decision that feels right for you and help you manage any discomfort that arises.

When I speak to new clients who struggle with this, I ask them if they could consider pausing the active pursuit of weight loss for a period of time. You have full body autonomy – you can always go back to the pursuit of weight loss if you wish. I don't condone this because of the reasons I have outlined in the previous chapter. Still, I am not living your life or walking in your shoes, so it's not my choice to make for you or for any of the people that I sit with in clinic, and it's certainly not my place to judge anyone who decides they would like to continue dieting. Putting a timeline on your decision to move away from dieting can help you take the first step if this dilemma paralyses you from taking any action.

Weight loss may or may not be a by-product of intuitive eating, but it is not and should not be used as a weight-loss tool. While intuitive eating does not align with dieting and intentional weight loss, that does not mean that intuitive eating is anti-weight loss. Some people will lose weight, some will gain weight, and some will stay the same. I have seen all three in clinic. Weight loss is not a prerequisite for success on an intuitive eating journey, and as a healthcare professional, I see all outcomes neutrally. Whether or not you lose or gain weight is unimportant to me. I am more interested in how a person feels and what they gain, other than weight, as they move through the process. You will reach your set point weight, the weight your body is healthiest and happiest at, when eating feels easy and effortless and you engage in consistent health-promoting behaviours, which we will cover in Part 3 of the book. Of course, your weight is influenced by certain lifestyle factors, such as the food you eat, how much exercise you do, and whether or not you engage in stress management and self-care techniques. You have influence but not control over your weight. By moving away from actively pursuing weight loss, you can begin to focus on the things you can control and will see long-term benefits from, like behaviour change. You are not a failure if your weight is over the 'healthy range'. Give yourself a break, do the best you can, and know that by engaging consistently with health-promoting behaviours, your weight will fall where it's meant to be.

What Is Positive Body Image?

What do the words 'positive body image' mean to you? If you were to imagine having a positive body image, what would that look like? Is there anyone in your life who you could say has a positive body image? If the answer to the last question is yes, then consider yourself lucky.

Body image is defined as how we feel about how we look and includes the feelings, thoughts, and perceptions one holds about their body. Therefore, it is the subjective picture one has of their own body, irrespective of how that body looks.[3] Positive body image is so much more than feeling good about your appearance. It matters just as much to appreciate how our bodies function, as well as how they look. We must acknowledge their unique characteristics, such as scars or blemishes. We hold a positive body image if we are able to appreciate a wide range of bodies outside the narrow beauty standard of popular media. We hold a positive body image if we are able to weather attacks on our body image, such as negative comments, or a lack of representation of our body type on Instagram. A positive body image is expressed through love for ourselves (i.e. self-care), but also love for others.[4]

Body image dissatisfaction is a complex construct that refers to negatively evaluating one's weight and shape. It impacts a wide range of individuals of all genders and can be seen in those with subclinical levels of disordered eating and those without eating disorders.[5]

Women of all ages report experiencing body image dissatisfaction, ranging from a low of 71.9 per cent in women aged 75 and above and up to 93.2 per cent of women between the ages of 25 and 34.[6] Research has shown that approximately 50 per cent of 13-year-old American girls reported being unhappy with their bodies. This number grew to nearly 80 per cent when girls reached 17 years of age.[7] This is not just a problem for younger women, with cohorts of women in their fifties showing relatively similar levels of body image dissatisfaction to women in their twenties, further supporting the theory that age is not a protective factor.[8] In clinic, I have seen body image dissatisfaction appear in people of all ages. A 2014 study found no significant difference in the rates of body image dissatisfaction for both American Caucasian and African American women, indicating that this problem exists beyond race.[9] There is also evidence to suggest that the recent pandemic may have exacerbated rates of body image dissatisfaction.[10] 'Normative discontent' is a term that has been used to describe the prevalence of body image dissatisfaction in women, outlining that this may have become a socially acceptable problem, which is understandable, given the long-standing historical focus on female body image.

Poor body image is commonly known to affect women; however, body image dissatisfaction is not just a female problem, despite being seen in broader society as a 'woman's issue'. If you identify as male and are reading this, I see you, and you are welcome here. The information in this chapter and the strategies I will share with you throughout will be helpful even if you don't identify as female.

Given that eating disorders affect women more than men, much of the research concerning eating disorders and body image is focused on female subjects. However, in a study of more than 50,000 adults, 41 per cent of men reported feeling too heavy and were self-conscious about their weight.[11] In a study of 6,187 boys aged 10 to 17, researchers found that one-third of participants reported weight concerns and that these increased consistently with age.[12]

Although body image dissatisfaction may manifest differently in men than women, the relative impact is similar. Poor body image is so prevalent: if you struggle with this, you're not alone. It can affect people of all shapes and sizes, but it can affect people more the further away they find themselves from the beauty ideal. I'm sure you had and perhaps still have some hang-ups about your own body if you've picked up this book and the statistics above are anything to go by. No person or group is immune to body image pressures. But although we cannot become immune to them, we can become more resilient and learn skills to validate our discomfort if and when it arises and learn to spiral up and out rather than deeper down into a body image disruption when it hits. This is where body image work comes in.

The Impact of Oppression

It wouldn't feel right to write a chapter on body image without spending some time talking about oppression and the impact this can have on the journey towards positive body image. Body image refers to the way we feel about our own bodies. Body-based oppression refers to the way the world we live in treats our bodies. Regarding the body, particular identities are often marginalized and oppressed in our culture – for example, in the case of fatness, blackness, or disability. Having one or more of these identities can provide you with extra challenges on the journey towards body acceptance. Since I do not have lived experience of any of these identities, I can't speak to what this is like, but I sit with people in clinic who do and have kindly shared their stories with me. It's important to acknowledge that no amount of loving oneself or accepting the body as it is will end the body-based oppression and discrimination that some people experience. For example, a thin, white, non-disabled person may experience negative body image but will not have to face discrimination in the doctor's office or on the street. A black, fat, disabled person may hold or be working towards a neutral, loving relationship with their own body but may still come up against body-based oppression, regardless of how much inner work they do on themselves and their body image. This is why the quest toward positive body image is not as simple as deciding to 'just love yourself'.

Body acceptance and neutrality are powerful tools to develop and work towards, liberating all people along the way. But body-based oppression must be tackled through a systemic shift where we all begin to uproot and challenge our biases. This can be difficult and downright uncomfortable for everyone involved, but without it, people will continue to suffer in ways they shouldn't have to. Many other people out there, primarily fat activists and authors like Aubrey Gordon, Da'Shaun L. Harrison, and others, can do this topic more justice than I ever could, so I recommend following, listening to, and reading the work of these people if you'd like to learn more. You will find a list of people I learn from at the end of this book.

The Importance of Body Image Work

Doing body image work is not about changing your body; the goal is to change how you *feel about* your body. Attempting to change your body is futile and maintaining weight loss over the long term is unattainable for most people. There is an analogy I often share with my clients to explain body image work and what it means to practise improving your body image. I believe that everyone can benefit from doing this work whether or not they fit into appearance ideals. Here's why.

Imagine jumping into your car and taking a solo trip from Dublin to Cork. For anyone who doesn't live in Ireland, this is about a three-hour drive spanning over 260 kilometres. The road consists of a motorway (or highway) for most of the journey. While on a long stretch of road, you get a flat tyre. There isn't a service station for miles. It's dark outside. You realize that you don't have a spare tyre and the tools needed to change it, or you don't have the skills to change a tyre because you've never had to and nobody has ever taught you. You're alone, and your phone is dead, so you can't call anyone. What do you do? You're pretty screwed, right? To get out of this situation, you will have to resort to potentially dangerous measures, like walking in the dark to the nearest service station or hitchhiking. This is what happens when you don't do body image work. You're left with few options to get out of a sticky situation. In the case of a body image disruption, this might look like embarking on a restrictive diet to attempt to change your body, which will lead to more harm and distress in the long-term.

Alternatively, imagine what it would feel like to have all the skills needed to change a tyre if you get a puncture. You have a spare, a jack, and a torch. You have a fully charged phone to google 'how to change a tyre' if you've never done it before. Doesn't it feel safer and more empowering? This is akin to the process of doing body image work. Doing the work and learning the skills will not prevent a flat tyre, but it will mean that you can deal with the situation, get back into your car, and move on. By doing body image work, the body image disruption is contained in the moment, rather than spilling out and bleeding into the rest of your life, affecting how you think, feel, and behave. It has less of an impact on your self-esteem and self-worth.

Positive body image is a lifelong journey, not a destination. This is because our bodies do not remain static throughout our lives. They constantly change over time, a process we cannot halt. There will be moments where the relationship between you and your body is under threat. This might come up during or after pregnancy, when you go through a life transition, age, or gain weight. Moving towards a positive body image is about internal acceptance rather than external changes. Doing body image work involves learning the coping skills required to self-regulate, self-soothe, and buffer against body image disruptions.

A body image disruption arises when you experience a situation that tests your relationship with your body — when the splitting of your identity occurs and you become the seer and the seen. This can happen when you see a photo of yourself, when you see your reflection in a mirror, when you are out shopping and nothing fits or looks good (we've all been there), or it can arise during life transitions such as break-ups or moving out of home, just to name a few. There are two ways you can react when you experience a body image disruption. You can spiral down deeper into the disruption and the uncomfortable emotions it brings, or you can spiral up and out of it. To do the latter, you must first validate your feelings and then employ a proactive coping strategy. When you learn how to do this, you begin to contain the body image disruption, resulting in a bad body image moment rather than a whole bad body image day. Without cultivating this skill, your feelings of insecurity about your body can begin to bleed into your day, your week, and your life and affect how you think, feel, and behave. You will remain vulnerable to the pressures from diet culture to change your body, and it will be difficult to buffer against these urges.

We shouldn't underestimate the power of doing body image work; it can truly change the trajectory of how you feel about yourself and your body. Your ability to deal with body image disruptions will only come with time and practice. Obtaining a positive body image is an active, not a passive, practice. It requires work, just like anything in life worth having, but it's worth it.

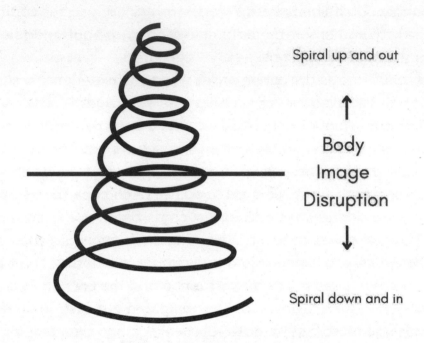

Spiral up and out

↑

Body
Image
Disruption

↓

Spiral down and in

Rebuilding Positive Body Image

I could probably write a whole book on rebuilding positive body image. Still, I'm going to give you some practical ways you can begin your journey towards respecting and accepting your here-and-now body. I use the term 'rebuilding' positive body image because, once upon a time, we all held an embodied relationship with ourselves, even if we can't remember it. Picture a small toddler on a beach, mucking around in the sand, sunscreen slathered in white patches over their whole body, hair stuck to their head with sweat but having a great time nonetheless. This is the picture of embodiment. OK, so being embodied doesn't have to look quite like this in adulthood, but you get my drift. To be embodied simply means to be connected to your body. When the embodiment we are all born with gets interrupted, we begin to see and judge ourselves from the outside — cue self-objecti-fication. To revisit Hillary McBride's analogy of self-objectification, being embodied means spending more time inside your house than out on your front lawn. From a toddler's perspective, their body allows them to play, explore, and have fun. They live fully inside their house, rather than standing outside on the lawn, judging themselves. Along the way, this connection with ourselves gets interrupted, and part of the journey back to positive body image is reconnecting with the embodied self.

When clients come to see me in clinic, they often say things like, 'I don't know if I can ever be OK with my body/being my current weight.' This can be a tough place to be, and if you feel like this, I am sorry. Your body is a beautiful container that carries you through life and allows you to experience all the good things life has to offer: hugging your loved ones, walking in nature, enjoying delicious food, travelling the world, or listening to the waves break on the beach. None of this would be possible without the body, so I hate how we as a society have been conditioned to abandon our bodies if they do not fit into an appearance ideal and evaluate them from the outside. Some people spend their whole lives hating their bodies, which is a sad thought.

The body image hierarchy is a tool I developed to support you if beginning to cultivate a positive body image seems like a momentous task that's somewhat out of reach, as it can feel for many of my clients. This hierarchy is based on Maslow's hierarchy of needs, a five-tier model of human needs. Needs lower down in the hierarchy must be satisfied before individuals can attend to needs higher up. This premise is the same for the body image hierarchy.

At the top of the body image hierarchy, we find body love. I think it's fair to say that we would all like to experience body love, and this is one of the elusive promises that diet culture lures us in with. However, attaining body love can seem too far out of reach, especially at the start of a body image journey. This is why we find body acceptance or neutrality one level below body love. Again, this can feel intangible for some people, so we must start at the bottom of the hierarchy by establishing body respect. Only when we have satisfied the needs of body respect do we begin to move up the hierarchy to the next level. Developing body respect is an excellent starting point, as there are concrete ways you can begin to do this.

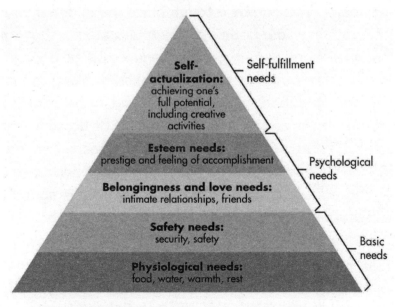

Maslow's Hierarchy of Needs

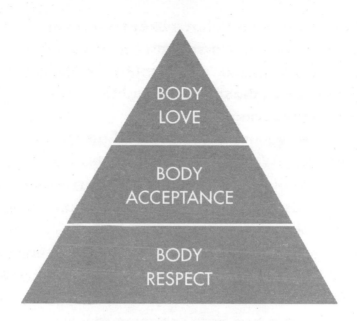

The Body Image Hierarchy

1. Redefine what beauty means to you
Beauty is a social construct: a very narrow idea of what is considered 'beautiful' has been created in our culture, giving rise to the beauty ideal. However, beauty is infinite; it is not a finite resource. It can be found everywhere and does not run out. One person's beauty does not take away from another's. Physical beauty can be found in many different shapes and sizes, we have just been led to believe that it can only be found in a thin body. This is not true. Redefining what it means to you is a powerful way of expanding the definition of beauty from an objective to a subjective perspective. Beauty truly is in the eye of the beholder, and by redefining your definition of beauty and seeking it out in your everyday life, you can begin to reshape

your own beliefs around what makes something or someone beautiful. You can begin doing this by looking out for simple displays of beauty in your environment – in the sun cracking through the clouds, the sound of laughter, or the blossoming of flowers in the spring.

Finding inner beauty in yourself and others will also help with this process. When you begin doing this, it may be easier to find inner beauty in others before finding it in yourself. Think about a few people in your life who you appreciate and admire. Is it because of their external beauty? I'm guessing not. It's probably because of how they make you feel, how you laugh and have fun in their company, how passionate they are about a particular topic or because they have a caring nature, to name a few. Here are some real-life examples of inner beauty that I see in my parents to show you how to do this (I will stop there to avoid hurting anybody due to exclusion since I have many more amazing people in my life – you know who you are).

My mam: honest, caring, authentic and goes above and beyond to help people in need.

My dad: strong-willed, trustworthy, fiercely proud and would do anything for his family.

When you begin to notice the inner beauty that emanates from the people you love, it will help you start doing this for yourself also. A simple way is to write down one thing you love about yourself every day in your journal. This needs to be practised consistently to make an impact. Push aside any ideas that doing this exercise means you 'have notions' about yourself. Self-love is powerful, and embracing it will go a long way in helping you to detach your self-worth from your external appearance.

2. Become adept at media literacy

Perhaps one of the most impactful ways to improve body image is to become critically aware of the content you are consuming from all forms of media, be it social media or mainstream media. Media literacy encourages us to ask questions about what we watch, hear and read. By becoming media-literate, you can begin to examine the messages behind the media you are exposed to and how it makes you feel about yourself and your own body. In turn, learning how to reject images and messages that could endanger body image will craft a media experience that protects rather than discourages positive body image. By following people of all shapes, sizes, colours, and abilities on social media, your definition of beauty will expand and broaden.

3. Build a body respect practice

The way we feel about our bodies is transient, and having a positive body image doesn't mean that you will never have bad body image moments. It simply means that you have more good days than bad days and that how you feel about your body doesn't dictate how you live your life. In these moments of struggle, having a body respect practice can make the difference between spiralling down and into a body image disruption or spiralling up and out of it. Likewise, engaging in body respect practices when you are feeling good can help protect you when you aren't. Here are a list of body respect practices you can begin to build into your life:

☐ Wearing underwear and clothes that fit you and feel comfortable

☐ Nourishing your body with food that makes you feel well

☐ Drinking enough water to hydrate your body

☐ Moving your body regularly in a way that feels joyful and not torturous

☐ Practising self-pleasure

☐ Massaging your body with body cream or oil

☐ Getting a professional massage

☐ Stretching your body

☐ Reminding yourself of your good qualities

☐ Stopping weighing yourself

☐ Eating intuitively by honouring hunger, fullness, and satisfaction cues (more on this in Part 2)

☐ Accepting your here-and-now body

☐ Journalling

☐ Being compassionate toward yourself

☐ Practising yoga and meditation

Undoing years, perhaps even decades, of built-up self-loathing towards your body is not something that can be achieved overnight, but you can decide to begin making more respectful and loving decisions towards yourself and your body right now. Once you decide that this is important to you, you can choose in each day, in each moment, to treat your body with the respect and love you deserve. At the beginning, this may seem like a foreign concept. It may feel clunky and difficult. Remember that with every single choice you are strengthening your decision to prioritize loving and respecting your body, and over time, it will become more and more natural.

But I Care About What I Look Like

This question comes up a lot with my clients: 'Am I allowed to care about what I look like?' My answer is always 'How could you not?' It is OK to care about your appearance. It's OK to want to look your best and pamper or dress yourself in a way that supports that. There is absolutely nothing wrong with this. If it makes you feel good, crack on! I love putting on a beautiful dress and a stunning pair of stilettos just as much as the next woman. I am not suggesting you need to get to a place where you do not care at all about what you look like. Caring about your appearance only becomes an issue when your worth is tied to what you look like on the outside or you make special efforts to look a certain way that takes energy from other areas of your life that you'd rather direct that energy to. Only you can determine if caring about your external appearance has gone too far. Ask yourself 'Would anything in my life change if I cared less about what I looked like on the outside?'

Do what makes you feel good. But know that you are enough, regardless of what you look like.

Affirmations

My worth is about so much more than a number on the scales.

I overcome body image challenges with ease because I am resilient and strong.

Every day I am becoming more resilient to diet culture messages.

I am so grateful for my body and all that it does for me.

I choose to respect my body.

I am learning to accept myself as I am.

Chapter 3:

The Power of Permission

Recently, a client told me that a large bar of chocolate had been sitting in her fridge for weeks. It was the first time this had happened in as long as she could remember. She was ecstatic and couldn't believe it. For so long, she honestly thought that she was addicted to food. She couldn't keep any 'treat' foods in the house, or she would eat them all until they were gone. She felt out of control. For years, she believed there was something wrong with her. Now, that Toblerone she'd bought at the airport was still sitting in the fridge, waiting to be enjoyed. Suddenly, she felt calm and in control. The chocolate didn't hold the same power over her as it had for so many years – decades even!

This is what happens when no food is off-limits. The power of permission surfaces as a result of giving yourself *unconditional* permission to eat all foods – that is, having no conditions attached to the food you eat.

Conditional permission looks like:

- ☐ Allowing yourself that slice of cake, but only after going to the gym

- ☐ Allowing yourself all foods, but only on certain days of the week

- ☐ Allowing your favourite foods, but only on cheat days

When *conditional* permission is attached to the food you eat, the control you wish to have over food will not materialize. If you want to be able to stop eating when full and always feel in control around all foods (yes, even the 'naughty' ones), then you must create the conditions required for the power of permission to surface.

I can't count how many times I've witnessed the power of permission surface with my clients; it's a big win when it happens. I do a little internal fist pump when people come into a session, their eyes twinkling with pride as they tell me they left food on their plate because they were full or wrapped up a share bag of crisps for later. That's because it doesn't just happen. It takes patience and bucketloads of self-trust. The point isn't to burn out on certain foods or never eat them again. The point is to allow all foods in unconditionally to make space for the power of permission to surface. When you give yourself unconditional permission to eat all foods, that's when the magic happens.

Diet culture teaches us that to be healthy we need to put controls on certain foods, or else we will overeat them. Trusting ourselves around food is something that diet culture has a vested interest in convincing us we cannot do. After all, the more out of control you feel around food, the more you feel like you need a diet to keep you in check, right? In reality, the more intense the restriction, the more intense the craving and the more intense the overeating. Dieting is based wholly and exclusively on restriction. To get to a place of feeling calm and in control around food, you need to go straight to the root of the issue and remove any restrictions you hold around food, giving yourself unconditional permission to eat. It's the only way. Giving yourself unconditional permission to eat looks like:

- ☐ Releasing any physical or mental restriction around food

- ☐ Allowing yourself to eat what you want, when you want

- ☐ Embracing food neutrality by releasing any binary or dichotomous language around food, such as labelling foods as 'good' or 'bad'

- ☐ Cultivating an abundance rather than a scarcity mindset around food

- ☐ Continuing to notice and reject diet mentality

Only when you give yourself unconditional permission to eat and have no restrictions around food will you be truly able to ask yourself, 'Do I want this food right now?' It's understandable if this feels scary for you — it's one of the most challenging aspects of the intuitive eating process for many, but it's a necessary part of the path to finding true food freedom.

Developing Self-Trust

A few years ago, I was being interviewed for a podcast and the host asked me a question that comes up every time I share the benefits behind the power of permission: 'All of this sounds great, but if I allow myself to eat whatever I want, won't I just eat pizza and chocolate all day long?' This is a common misconception about intuitive eating, and it may well happen at the beginning of the intuitive eating process, which we refer to as the honeymoon phase. But what do you imagine would happen if you ate pizza and chocolate at every meal, for two weeks straight? You'd probably get sick of it eventually, and start craving some more variety, right?

The honeymoon phase can be very liberating, freeing, and empowering, but for some, it may also feel a little bit out of control. When you begin allowing in foods that have been restricted, either physically or mentally, for a very long time, there is a high likelihood that you will go a little batshit crazy on these foods. This is a normal and expected part of the process. I would argue that it's an essential part of the process. But, just like any honeymoon phase, it doesn't last forever. When you are in the throes of eating pizza every night or polishing off a tub of Ben & Jerry's a few times a week, this can be difficult to accept, especially if you have a fear of weight gain, which most people do. After all, that's why you probably started dieting in the first place, right? You've probably been told (and subsequently believed) that you must contain your insatiable appetite and animalistic tendencies around food by restricting certain foods, or you will continue to lose control over your weight.

You may even have personally experienced this over and over again, which only confirmed this belief. But please trust me when I tell you that this is not true. Restriction, aka dieting, causes this feeling of being out of control around food. You are not broken. You are experiencing the effects of restriction and diet culture. When my clients struggle with believing they will one day feel in control around all foods, my job is to be their anchor before they can be the anchor for themselves. And although you may not be working closely with me, as you read this book, I want to be your anchor, too, by reassuring you that this honeymoon phase will not last forever for you either. Over time, you can become your own anchor through developing self-trust. This will be your saviour. You are in a relationship with your body, and the trust between you and your body has been broken.

When you start a diet, some specific rules and regulations must be adhered to. For example, one of those rules may be to restrict 'treat' foods during the week and only to allow yourself to have them at the weekend. When you get a craving during the week for chocolate, cake, or takeaway, for example, this goes against the diet rule, so you don't allow yourself to have it. You deny the craving. This may happen repeatedly; the more 'willpower' you have, the more you deny yourself. Until that fateful day when you say 'screw it' and eat the cake. Sound familiar? Each time you adhere to the diet rule, regard-less of the craving or needs of your body, the trust between you both erodes a little bit more.

I have an online course and group coaching programme about the foundations of intuitive eating, and I asked those in the group if they could count how many times they have denied a craving or followed a diet rule, rather than attending to the needs of their body. I gave them four options: 0–25, 25–50, 50–100, or over 100 times. They said it was well over 100 times. That's over 100 times the trust between them and their bodies has been broken. That trust needs to be rebuilt; and rebuilding trust takes time and commitment.

You are rebuilding trust with your body every time you allow yourself food that hasn't been freely permitted in the past. To further understand this concept, let's apply it to relationships. When one person breaks the trust of another, either once or many times, it will take time and commitment before that trust returns. The person who has broken the trust of another will need to show up consistently by behaving in specific ways before the betrayed person will feel as though they can trust again. Every instance of doing as they say they will is important and makes a difference. It's the same with food. From now on, I'd like you to think of yourself as being in a relationship with your body, and just like any happy relationship, trust is an integral part of that. You have the capacity to rebuild this self-trust piece by piece every time you honour the needs of the body.

Restriction and How It Manifests

There are two types of restriction – physical restriction and mental restriction. Both forms have an equal impact on increased cravings and, subsequently, overeating, which can make you feel out of control around food.

The dieting pendulum is a concept developed by psychologist and HAES (Health At Every Size) founder Deb Burgard to explain what happens when restrictions are placed on food. Imagine a pendulum that has been pulled back as far as possible. This is what Deb refers to as dietland, where there are a lot of rules and rigidities around food. Now, we all know that nobody can stay in dietland forever, just like a pendulum can't be pulled back forever. When you let go of that pendulum, it will swing over to the opposite side, into donutland, where eating may feel uncomfortable and uncontrollable. The only way to return to balance, where eating feels flexible and fluid, is to stop pulling the pendulum back into dietland. In other words, restriction and rigidity around food needs to be removed. A large part of my role as a food therapist at the beginning of someone's journey is to help them get through this process. I hold onto them (metaphorically) for dear life and hope that they won't be pulled back to dietland.

THE DIETING PENDULUM

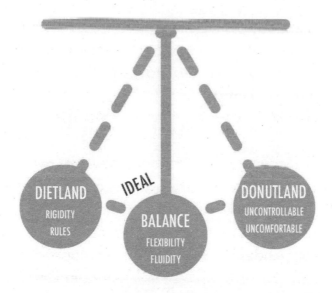

A common question that I get from my clients is, 'I've been allowing all foods in for months, but I'm still overeating or bingeing. What am I doing wrong?' Most people will manage to release physical restriction, but will still be mentally restricting. Physical restriction is a little easier to spot, whereas spotting and removing mental restriction requires a bit more work. Removing physical restriction can be seen as a behavioural shift, whereas removing mental restriction requires a mental and emotional shift: they require different skills.

Physical restriction looks like:

☐ Not allowing in certain foods or food groups (for reasons other than medical, ethical and so on)

☐ Only allowing certain foods on specific days of the week

☐ Saying no to a food when you really want to say yes

Mental restriction looks like:

☐ Allowing yourself to eat all foods, but only a certain quantity

☐ Allowing yourself to eat all foods, but only when you're hungry

☐ Feeling guilty about eating certain foods

☐ Labelling foods as good and bad

☐ Judging your food choices

☐ Blaming food for your weight

If your mouth says yes, but your mind says no, the deprivation effect will persist and you will continue to feel out of control around food. Diet mentality can be buried deeply within the mind. When the hooks of mental restriction are still deeply embedded and there is no effort to try and remove them, the honeymoon phase will not end. How can you be free if you are still shackled to old and faulty food beliefs? Holding onto these beliefs around food may make you feel safe and protected from being out of control around food. In reality, they are causing this loss of control because they encourage a scarcity mindset and communicate that restriction is coming. It's time to let them go. You can do this by embracing an abundance mindset around food, calling out binary thinking and cultivating food neutrality.

It takes time to reprogram the mind — this is not something that happens overnight. However, the more you practise, the more this new mindset is being laid down in the psyche. Every single instance where you embrace abundance over scarcity or cultivate food neutrality is having an effect, even if it doesn't feel like it in the moment.

The Habituation Effect

Do you feel addicted to food or like you can't stop eating once you start? Do you experience intense cravings and do everything in your power not to give in to them? If so, a lack of habituation might be the problem, not food addiction.

A few years ago, I packed my bags and spent Christmas and New Year on holiday in Sri Lanka. It's an amazing place with pillow-soft sand, jungle yoga shalas and incredible mountain views. The one thing it doesn't have is good choc-olate – there wasn't a Cadbury's bar in sight! The trip was only two weeks long, but I started to crave chocolate about a week in. I found myself stopping at corner shops to check in case they had any chocolate I recognized. I tried some of the local varieties, but none of them hit the spot (that's being kind). I realized how much my mind had become consumed with the quest of finding some chocolate to satisfy the craving. I wasn't intentionally restricting chocolate, but it was restricted nonetheless. I knew what was happening and could watch my reaction to the inability to satisfy the need; it was fascinating to observe. This restriction was leading to the obsessing over chocolate and it became more intense as the days went on, until I found myself in the taxi to the airport to catch my flight back to Dublin.

I started dreaming about the large Toblerone mini bags you can get in the duty free – you know the ones with all the different flavours? The excitement was palpable and continued until I hit Abu Dhabi airport. I sauntered into the duty free, picked up one of the (massive) bags and went on to find a good spot to relax before my flight with the chocolate, a coffee, and my book in tow. The first thing I noticed as I began to enjoy the chocolate was how incredible it tasted. Now, I've eaten Toblerone many, many times before, but I couldn't remember it tasting *this* good. The second thing I noticed was that it was taking quite a lot of chocolate to feel satisfied. I was eating much more than I usually would. This continued right up until I landed in Dublin – I couldn't get enough of that damn Toblerone!

This was the result of being restricted for just two weeks.

I don't restrict any food, ever; I allow myself free rein with chocolate in my day-to-day life. As a result, it's not that exciting to me and, yes, I eat it multiple times a week, but it's rare that I overeat it to the point of feeling uncomfortable, lethargic, or unwell. So in just two short weeks, I was beginning to see the impact of having *unintentionally* restricted chocolate. I'm a nutritionist, who does this for a living. I have all the knowledge, tips, and tricks in the book. I sit with people every day helping them to rebuild their relationship with food and body image. I have a very healthy relationship with food. I have spent over a decade continuously studying and working in this area of health, not to mention investing in my own therapy and inner work, and I was not immune to the impact of restriction.

The only way to protect yourself from this is to work towards habituating with all foods, and habituation cannot occur alongside restriction. Removing restrictions is the secret to feeling in control around all foods. Ironically, you need to release control to get control back. This is not just based on anecdotal experience I've had with clients: it's rooted in science.

In science, habituation is a form of learning in which repeated exposure to a stimulus leads to a decreased response. Repeated exposure is a necessary element of this process to reach habituation. Scientists studying the long-term habituation response randomly assigned 'obese' and 'non-obese' women to receive macaroni and cheese either once a week for five weeks or daily for one week. In both 'obese' and 'non-obese' women, daily presentation of the same food resulted in faster habituation and less energy intake than did once-weekly presentation of food. Note that they found that there was a reduced energy intake — not an increased energy intake. As I explained before, after the initial honeymoon phase, the habituation response results in people eating less, not more of the restricted food.

It takes less time to habituate to a food when it has the same characteristics, such as brand and flavour.[1] So when you begin adding back in food that has previously been restricted, it's a good idea to focus on one particular food (and flavour) at a time — for example, Cadbury's Dairy Milk — and add it into your meals or snacks every day. I know what you're thinking — 'Doesn't this go against all the advice I've ever received around food?!' Probably. But has any advice you've received to restrict or cut out certain foods or food groups, or remove them from your home, actually worked? Or does it just result in you obsessing about them more? The goal for this stage is habit-uation, not healthy eating. We can get to that later, but you can't truly embrace healthy eating without feeling in control first. Otherwise, you will always be desiring 'unhealthy' food and rejecting 'healthy' food, because the 'unhealthy' food has been put on a pedestal. I'll bet that foods you have categorized as 'healthy' haven't been put up on a pedestal in the same way chocolate, crisps, and cake have. Tell me, do you ever feel out of control around broccoli? If the answer is yes, then I need to hear from you immediately! Hit me up on Instagram — @nutri-tionwithniamh. Most people laugh when I ask this question and say 'Of course not!' Of course you don't, because broccoli more than likely hasn't been restricted.

When I start working with someone new, I ask them if there are any foods aound which they feel completely safe. No one has ever said chocolate, crisps, or cake — 99 per cent of the time people answer fruit and vegetables or diet foods that have been freely allowed, such as low-fat yoghurt. Now, if this doesn't prove that there's a problem with restriction, I don't know what will. It's not a coincidence that the only foods most people feel completely in control around are those that haven't been branded as 'bad'. I've put 'healthy' and 'unhealthy' in inverted commas because these labels encourage binary thinking and have a flavour of categorizing foods as good and bad about them, which brings us onto our next point.

Embracing Food Neutrality

'I've been so bad this week.'

'Chocolate is so bad for me.'

'I should only eat good foods.'

'I must be good this week since I was so bad at the weekend.'

'I am only eating healthy food this week.'

These are all phrases I hear regularly out in the world. I'm sure you have too or have said some of these yourself. We cannot underestimate the power of the meanings attached to food through the language we use to describe it. Judgement and shame have no place in rebuilding your relationship with food. Shame does not make you do better. How can you achieve food freedom if you feel shame about doing some-thing so basic as eating? When I began studying nutritional science at the tender age of seventeen, I remember sitting in a lecture, learning about dietary guidelines. These are exactly that: guidelines. They shouldn't be taken as hard-and-fast rules. But when certain foods are categorized as good or bad, as they can be when these guidelines are communicated, it can elicit feelings of judgement and shame. I remember feeling like a fraud sitting in that lecture, since I was learning that foods like chocolate, crisps, biscuits and so on 'should not be eaten every day' and here I was, eating these foods more regularly than was recommended. This is when I began to feel judgement and shame, as if this behaviour was something I should hide from others — especially as I was studying to become a nutritionist. Now, of course it's not conducive to health and well-being for these foods to make up a large proportion of your diet. However, labelling these foods as 'bad' is not the answer.

There is no such thing as good and bad foods. We need to be aware of the subconscious messages we are sending to ourselves and others when we use binary language around food — good vs bad, healthy vs unhealthy, clean vs indulgent. When we use descriptors such as 'bad' to describe certain foods, it can result in food guilt. You feel guilt when you believe you have done something wrong. Eating food is not wrong. You are not a bad person because you ate some chocolate. The food guilt you experience when you eat a food labelled as 'bad' pushes you to restrict and, as a result, it sets the binge—restrict cycle in motion. Hello, dieting pendulum. To free yourself of this cycle, you need to rewrite the narrative and remove any binary language or judgement about food.

Any-time you catch yourself using any of the following:

- ☐ Good
- ☐ Bad
- ☐ Unhealthy
- ☐ Indulgent
- ☐ Guilt-free
- ☐ Processed
- ☐ Junk
- ☐ Treat
- ☐ Dirty
- ☐ Cheat meal
- ☐ Guilty pleasure

replace them with:

- ☐ Play food
- ☐ Soul food
- ☐ Nourishing
- ☐ Nutritious
- ☐ Nutrient-rich
- ☐ Breakfast

- ☐ Lunch

- ☐ Dinner

- ☐ Snack

- ☐ Tasty

- ☐ Delicious

- ☐ Satisfying

- ☐ Hearty

Or just plain call it what it is: chocolate, fruit, bread, and so on. There is no need to attach a judgement to food, since this keeps you further disconnected from the self and attached to the narrative that the food you eat determines whether you are a good or bad person.

Abundance vs Scarcity

It's a normal human response to want something more when you know you can't have it. Even if we don't really want something, the minute it becomes scarce, we panic and begin to feel that we do indeed want that thing. When something — anything — is freely available, it becomes less exciting. Let's circle back to the lockdowns of 2020 and 2021 due to the coronavirus pandemic. I know, I know, nobody wants to remember this time — but stay with me. Do you remember what it felt like to not have any freedom? Do you remember how we all took our freedom for granted before it was taken away from us? No nights out. No meeting friends for dinner or drinks. No meeting new people. No dancing with random strangers on a dance floor. No travel. No hugs from your family. No chats by the water cooler in work. It was rough and something I hope we never have to experience again. Now, do you remember how badly you wanted to do all of these things once they were taken away? When these things were freely available and you could do them whenever you wanted, I'm guessing you didn't even pay them a second thought. This is the power of abundance vs scarcity. I'm sure you still enjoy doing all of these things, but I'm guessing there's less urgency to do them now, since you know there is less likelihood they will be taken away from you. Scarcity leads to increased desire; abundance leads to decreased desire.

It's perfectly acceptable, important even, to desire and receive pleasure from food, but it's not good for that desire to control you, which is what can happen when there is a sense of scarcity with food. Unfortunately, many people in the world experience food poverty, but most of you who have picked up this book will be privileged enough to have ample access to food. If this is the case, you can begin to embody an abundance mindset around food through observing and reframing your thoughts. Here are some examples:

Scarcity mindset: I don't know when this food will be available again, so I better eat as much as I can now.

Abundance mindset: This food will always be available to me.

Scarcity mindset: I really shouldn't eat this food; it's so unhealthy.

Abundance mindset: I am allowing myself to have all

foods, without guilt.

Scarcity mindset: I shouldn't keep chocolate in the house or I will eat it all.

Abundance mindset: I will keep all foods in the house and doing this will help me to eventually feel in control, knowing I can have them whenever I want.

Scarcity mindset: I can have this food, but only a certain quantity.

Abundance mindset: I am placing no restrictions on this food and can eat until I feel satisfied, knowing that I can always have more later.

The more you nurture this mindset of abundance, the less power and control certain foods will have over you and the closer you will get to food freedom.

Troubleshooting Overeating

If you are going through the honeymoon period right now and you are finding it challenging, I want to reassure you that overeating during this time on foods that have been previously restricted is an entirely normal and expected part of the process. I know how hard this can be, but it's an essential part of rebuilding your relationship with food so that you can get to a place of peace and control around all foods. Your body is simply responding physiologically and psychologically to scarcity. You can, however, ensure that the conditions are right to prevent as much overeating as possible. Please keep in mind that even when these conditions are in place, it's expected to overeat previously restricted foods while you habituate to them. The only way out of this period is through — there are no short-cuts. In the meantime, ask yourself the following questions:

1. Time: Are you eating regularly enough, i.e. every three to four hours?

2. Quantity: When you eat, are you eating enough to satisfy hunger?

3. Variety: Are you eating a variety of foods and food groups?

4. Restriction: Are you still either physically or mentally restricting any foods?

If you answer no to any of the questions from one to three and yes to question four, try to implement the conditions described in that question and see if that helps. If you answer yes to questions one to three and no to question four, then you are supporting yourself well as you navigate the honey-moon period. When you get to question four, be really honest with yourself. Remember that mental restriction will have just as much impact on you as a physical restriction. Are you secretly mentally restricting? Are you allowing all previously restricted foods in but with sneaky control strategies such as limiting the quantity of them? If so, this is conditional permis-sion, and the deprivation effect will persist. I know that this is challenging — it's quite possibly the most difficult period of rebuilding your relationship with food — but the sooner you let go of these restrictions, the sooner you will reach food freedom. If you are really struggling with this and you feel stuck in the honeymoon period, as many of my clients have in the past, reach out for professional support if you can. It may be that something else is keeping you stuck here. Having professional support can be the difference between drowning in this period or learning how to swim out of it.

But What about My Health?

People often grapple with this question when they find themselves in the honeymoon period, where they may be eating a lot of foods that have been on their naughty list for quite some time. You might be thinking, 'This can't be healthy?' To explore this further, let's revisit the definition of health. The World Health Organization (WHO) defines health as a 'state of complete physical, mental, and social wellbeing and not merely the absence of disease and infirmity'. Health is so much more than what you put into your mouth. We need to expand the definition of what we mean when we use the word 'healthy'.

When people come to work with me, either in a one-to-one capacity or through any of my online programmes, some of their primary goals are often to obsess less over food and regain control over their eating behaviours. They tell me there's a little voice in their head that judges every food choice and is constantly criticizing them when they don't make the 'right' ones. They tell how they've missed out on many social occasions and their unhealthy relationship with food or their body affects their relationships with friends, family, and partners. They describe a lack of presence when they do spend time with people they love. Perhaps you can also identify with some of these reasons. Do you think any of these experiences align with the WHO's definition of health? An unhealthy relationship with food doesn't affect just your physical health but also your mental and social health, as can be seen in these real-life examples. When this question comes up in clinic, I like to use the 'zooming out' strategy. This is where we try to look at the bigger picture and check in with the overall goal. The end goal right now is a healthy relationship with food. We're playing the long game here, and to heal from all of the above examples of disease I've mentioned, we may need to put in place some strategies that, in the interim, seem counter-intuitive but are essential to the healing process. Yes, we are allowing all foods in without restriction, but we are doing so with intention.

This is not a checking-out process; it's a checking-in process, to heal from the restriction that has affected your physical, mental, and social health. We are checking in with ourselves throughout the experience of eating these foods, by attuning to hunger, fullness, and satisfaction cues. Instead of checking out completely while eating these foods, we are checking in and asking ourselves:

- ☐ Am I hungry and if so, will this food satisfy me?

- ☐ How does this food taste?

- ☐ How does this food feel in my body?

- ☐ Would I choose to eat this way again?

- ☐ Would I need less or more of this food next time to feel satisfied?

When you do this, it will give you ample information about yourself that will contribute towards the big picture of rebuilding your relationship with food. We are doing this now so that one day, in the future, you will be able to eat all foods with ease and control and to awaken the intuitive eater so you can choose foods that make your body feel well. Not because you've been told you have to, but because you want to. Once you trust that the foods that have been previously restricted will be there for you if you want them in an hour, or tomorrow, or the next day, or next week, you can finally listen to the messages of your body and only eat enough of them to make you feel satisfied, both from a taste and body perspective (more on how to tune into this in Chapter 7). This is all in the name of long-term, sustainable health.

Affirmations

I embrace abundance over scarcity.

I trust that the honeymoon period is temporary.

Every day I am closer to feeling more in control around food.

I release all physical and mental restrictions around food.

I prioritize the rebuilding of self-trust.

I trust the process.

Chapter 4:

Uncovering the Inner Critic

Do you have a voice inside your own mind that berates you or tells you you're not good enough? As I sit down for the umpteenth time to write the book you are holding in your hands, I start hearing a voice in my head that says:

'How do you know what you're writing is even any good?'

'You're never going to finish this book by the deadline.'

'What will people think?'

'You should just back out now before exposing yourself to any judgement.'

This is the voice of the inner critic. Writing a book may be romanticized, but in reality it's extremely difficult, and since it's a new challenge, it's prime fuel for the voice of my inner critic to increase in volume. You may hear this voice when you make a mistake, start a new job, do something for the first time, such as entering a new gym or exercise class, or when learning how to drive. When you try something new or attempt to change a pattern that's been there for a long time – perhaps an unhealthy relationship with food – the inner critic will often come into the spotlight. It can be a right old thorn in your side and we all have one.

The inner critic shouts negative barbs and its output is often described as automatic negative thoughts. It's the voice that says you're not good enough as you are and that you need to fix or change yourself. It can prevent you from taking the steps needed to do something or change something you desperately want to in your life. Ironically, the inner critic has developed to protect you from danger and keep you safe. Its original purpose is to ensure your survival. Even though where you find yourself right now might be painful and unsustainable, at least it's familiar; 'better the devil you know than the devil you don't', right? What's familiar is comfortable. Change is hard because uncertainty is difficult for us to contend with, but uncertainty is a non-negotiable part of growth. Unfortunately, in the process of trying to keep you safe, your inner critic cuts you off from opportunities that allow you to grow and evolve if it's left unchecked and unmanaged. Fear ends up running the show.

The inner critic usually develops in childhood and it can be a learned behaviour from parents or caregivers. If you grow up with critical parents, these words can become internalized within the psyche. One of my clients who struggled with her inner critic said it resembled the criticisms she received from her parents around food and her body as a child. Since these criticisms started in early childhood, when her unconscious beliefs were formed, it took her quite some time to detach from them, and they still crop up when she is feeling vulnerable or threatened. For her, the inner critic sounds like:

'You shouldn't eat that food. It's so bad for you.'

'No one will ever love you if you're fat.'

'You need to lose weight or you'll get bullied in school.'

I know. Pretty horrific. I have many clients with thoughts that resemble the above; maybe they resonate with you too. The inner critic can be extremely harsh and most of us would never speak to a friend the way we speak to ourselves. To get an insight into your own inner critic, pay attention to this harsh voice. Is it speaking to you in the first person or otherwise? For example, is this voice saying something like 'You won't succeed' or 'You won't be happy if you don't lose weight'? If so, it's not your voice. It's one that has been projected onto you. Can you identify who owns this voice? Is it the voice of a parent, caregiver, or someone else from your past? Or is it the voice of diet-culture messaging at large? Try to find the origin of your inner critic. This will help when you begin to challenge it and take back control. You do not want your inner critic driving the bus.

Uncovering the inner critic and removing it from having power over you is an important part of finding food and body image freedom. The inner critic can keep you stuck in food and body image obsession by telling you that the only way you can be successful, desirable, healthy, happy, and so on is if you are in a thinner body. It can maintain beliefs that you have internalized from diet culture around food and your body. If you believe this voice, and it's granted the driver's seat in your life, it will inhibit you from freeing yourself from diet culture. You *can* take back control from this voice. You can get to a place where you feel at peace with food and your body, where eating is easy and effortless.

If this were to happen for you, what would you do with your day, your week, your year, your life? For many people that I have worked with, their struggles with food and their body have held them back in life. Freeing yourself from this requires uncovering and challenging the inner critic. Challenging the inner critic not only helps with rebuilding a healthy relationship with food, but it will also have a positive impact on the rest of your life. For the purposes of this book, we will be focusing mainly on how it relates to food and body image, but know that the strategies discussed in this chapter will help to alleviate the hold your inner critic has over you, no matter the subject.

Becoming Aware of Your Inner Critic

In one of my favourite books, *The Untethered Soul*, the author, Michael Singer, speaks about getting to know your inner roommate.[1] The incessant chatter inside your head is this inner roommate who never seems to give you a moment's peace. Taming your inner roommate is an important step towards freeing yourself from the influence of this running dialogue on your life.

A lot of the journey towards freeing yourself from the inner critic is about becoming aware of your thoughts. Observing your mind and creating separation between you and your thoughts is key to developing self-awareness. Your inner critic is a compilation of thoughts from inside your mind. Just because you have a thought doesn't mean it's true. Taking every thought as true is a risky business. Letting your mind take the wheel is like being taken on a dangerous joyride with a drunk driver. Remember that the inner critic has developed to keep you safe, but it doesn't always have your personal growth in mind. Rather than immediately acting on a thought, take a breath, become aware of it, and ask yourself 'Is this thought true? Or is it a reaction based on a past experience?' Sometimes your thoughts will tell you that it's not safe to move away from dieting or the pursuit of intentional weight loss. Or that you need to look a certain way to belong and be accepted. These thoughts are a product of diet culture. They keep you small and locked out of realizing that you are enough, just as you are, right now in this moment. You deserve love and respect, and the right people will give that to you. If you let the thoughts of the inner critic run the show, you'll find yourself in that car with the drunk driver. And that's a dangerous place to be.

When I was twenty-three, I went to my first yoga class. It was there that I learned how to observe my mind from afar. It was life-changing. Suddenly, I realized I didn't have to listen to every crazy thought my mind gave me because they were just thoughts. Thinking something doesn't make it true. Yoga and meditation are some of the best ways to learn how to become aware of your thoughts and, therefore, your inner critic. I have recorded a short meditation and included it as part of the book tools to help you with this. Navigate nutritionwithniamh.com and download it to get started with observing your thoughts.

Thinking Traps

I see several thinking traps come up a lot with my clients while on the journey of rebuilding a healthy relationship with food and body image. These cognitive distortions can wreak havoc if they're allowed to run the show. If these thinking traps show up in your own mind, it gives you a perfect opportunity to practise your self-compassion skills which I will speak more about later on in this chapter. Respond to them with compassion and rationality.

All-or-nothing thinking

When you engage in all-or-nothing thinking, also known as black-and-white thinking, you evaluate your life in extreme terms: you're either all in or all out. When you think in these dichotomous terms, all-or-nothing behaviours follow, such as:

☐ Being really 'good' or really 'bad'

☐ On a food plan or off a food plan

☐ Either eating no 'treats' or only eating 'treats'

Perfectionistic thinking

This is where everything is either perfect or it's a disaster. Perfectionistic thinking is an extension of all-or-nothing thinking. I see this a lot with my clients, since they are often the kind of people who are dedicated and committed. Unfortunately, for many of these people, and maybe for you too, this can come with a side of perfectionism — the refusal to accept anything less than perfect. For example:

If I don't eat perfectly, I am a failure.

If I don't lose weight, I have failed.

There's no point in doing anything if it's not done perfectly.

To resolve all-or-nothing and perfectionistic thinking, you must embrace the grey. This is something I talk about a lot in my practice. There is no such thing as a perfect diet or a perfect relationship with food. It doesn't exist. These thinking traps don't allow for the messy nuance of your relationship with food and how both your internal and external circumstances impact it. Embrace the grey with open arms.

Catastrophizing
Catastrophizing occurs when you believe the worst is going to happen. This can get you into a real muddle and leave you feeling miserable as a result. When you get caught in this thinking trap, you may fixate on the worst possible outcome and treat it as likely, even when it is not. When it comes to rebuilding your relationship with food and body image, this thinking trap affirms the belief that your happiness, health, and self-worth are dependent upon your body size or shape (hello there, diet culture, my old friend). It may manifest in thoughts such as:

I am always going to feel like this.

I'll never find a partner with this body.

If I don't lose weight, I will be unhealthy and die early.

Using affirmations, such as the ones sprinkled throughout this book, and continuing to use the reframing technique we spoke about in Chapter 1 will help to offset this form of negative self-talk.

Developing Your Inner Friend

Developing an inner friend as an antidote to the inner critic is based on the concept of the inner child. We all have an inner child that is triggered when we experience situations that remind us of certain feelings that we could not process or understand as a small child – the unhealed hurts we have picked up along the way. The source of the inner critic is the wounded inner child. These wounds come from our earliest experiences of feeling less than or unworthy. If the inner critic is trying to protect you and keep you safe, the inner friend is that part of you that is strong, wise, and knows that, whatever happens, you can handle it. It speaks to you with compassion and empathy.

Cultivating an inner friend can help to calm the inner critic, rather than letting it take over and dictate your thoughts, feelings, and behaviour. I like to think of the inner friend as having collected experiences and wisdom that can reassure the inner critic that everything is in hand. Rather than demonizing the inner critic and trying to fight it, you can meet it with compassion and remember why it has developed: to keep you safe. By befriending the inner critic, you acknow-ledge this and thank it for its good intentions, but ultimately, you have final say as to whether you follow its advice or not. The inner critic is fuelled by fear and those fears need to be met with self-compassion. By using self-compassion, you can begin to strengthen the voice of the inner friend and weaken the voice of the inner critic. Without honing this skill, we can all fall victim to the inner critic and the fear it is built upon will end up driving the bus. Here are some examples of how the inner friend might respond to the inner critic, as it relates to food and body image:

Inner critic: Your body is so disgusting.
Inner friend: Your body is a beautiful container that carries you through life and allows you to experience the wonderful things it has to offer.

Inner critic: No one will ever love you if you're fat.
Inner friend: You are so much more than your body. You deserve to be loved for more than your external appearance.

Inner critic: You're never going to 'get' intuitive eating. Food will always have a hold over you.
Inner friend: Anything worth having takes time. You are getting closer to food freedom every day.

Inner critic: If it's not perfect, then you're a failure. You can never do anything right so you may as well not even try.
Inner friend: We are approaching every experience with curiosity instead of judgement. Every experience has something to teach you. There is no such thing as perfect.

Self-Compassion: The Antidote

Self-compassion is extending compassion to oneself in instances of perceived inadequacy, failure, or general suffering. It is the most effective antidote to the inner critic and underpins all other techniques. Without self-compassion, any other method to offset the inner critic can fall short. When you feel unhappy with yourself or your body, self-compassion is crucial. When you experience a body image disruption, the immediate response can be the urge to fix the body, respond with punishment or restriction and be further dragged into the need to control your food and exercise routine. Unfortunately, this can lead to more problems being created than fixed. Remember that the inner critic is trying to keep you safe, based on what diet culture has taught you. It says, 'You need to diet to control your weight and shape and always be on high alert for gaining weight. You should do everything in your power to prevent this from happening.' However, doing this keeps you stuck, feeling trapped and out of control around food and brings you further away from food freedom. Removing the inner critic from the driver's seat and replacing it with self-compassion is integral to feeling free from food and body image struggles.

Kristin Neff has defined self-compassion as being composed of three main elements: mindfulness, common humanity and self-kindness.

1. Mindful awareness vs over-identification: observing thoughts and feelings as they are, without

trying to suppress or deny them, rather than over-identifying with them and getting swept away by negative reactivity.

2. Common humanity vs isolation: recognizing that suffering is a universal experience rather than something that happens to you alone.

3. Self-kindness vs self-judgement: being warm and understanding towards ourselves when we suffer, fail, or feel inadequate rather than ignoring our pain or flagellating ourselves with self-criticism.[2]

How Would You Treat a Friend?

Another way to look at cultivating self-compassion is to consider how you would treat a friend if they were in a similar situation. You may not feel worthy of self-compassion, or you may feel like you need some tough love to 'get your act together'. Very often, we treat ourselves differently than we treat others. The words you say to yourself have just as much impact on you as they would if they came from another person. Most of us would never speak to a friend the way we speak to ourselves, which is why thinking about how you would treat a friend if they were struggling with a similar situation can help you access self-compassion.

Many of my clients struggle with self-compassion, but cultivating this in response to inadequacy or suffering is just like any other skill: we need to practise to improve. When we feel low or vulnerable, the inner critic gets louder and can take over our thoughts, feelings and behaviour. This is when we need self-compassion most, but when it's also difficult to access. In one of the group calls within my online course and group coaching programme, 'The Foundations of Intuitive Eating', I asked the attendees the following questions and gave them some time to journal on them:

1. How do you treat yourself when you struggle with food or body image? How do you speak to your-self? Is the tone harsh or kind?

2. What would you say to a friend if they struggled with the same issue? Is the tone harsh or kind?

It was an eye-opening exercise for them. They told me how their answers to each question were completely different. When they themselves were struggling, their inner voice was harsh and critical, but when a friend was struggling, they were kind and compassionate. This showed them all that they did indeed have the capability to be compassionate – they just needed to turn that compassion towards themselves. If their answers resonate with you too, it can be helpful to imagine a friend providing the compassion that you need in your times of struggle. You can do this through the meditation below (or you can download an audio version from my website nutritionwithniamh.com).

Compassionate friend meditation
Come to a comfortable position. You can be sitting up or lying down, whatever feels most comfortable. Gently close your eyes, or if that feels very uncomfortable, turn your gaze

down towards the earth. Take a few deep breaths in through the nose and out through the mouth. In through the nose, and out through the mouth. And one more time, in through the nose, and out through the mouth. Place both hands on your heart. Commit to gifting yourself some loving kindness over the next few minutes. Your only priority is to focus on yourself. Now begin to connect with the breath in the body, breathing deeply into the belly. Feel the breath travel in through the nose and down into the belly and the chest. Breathe deeply into the belly. Feel the belly and the chest rise on the inhale and fall on the exhale. Now bring to mind one of your favourite places. It could be a room in your house, your favourite chair, or a place you've visited in your past. Make yourself comfortable here and bring to mind all of the details of your favourite place. In the distance, you see a figure approaching you. As they get closer, they ask if they can sit down beside you. This person embodies the qualities of wisdom, strength, warmth, and unconditional accept-ance. You feel completely safe and supported in their presence. It could be a compassionate person from your past or your present or it could just be a kind, loving pres-ence, without any particular name or form. Invite this being to take a seat beside you. Enjoy the feeling of their loving presence. See this compassionate friend in your mind's eye. There is nothing you need to do other than to enjoy their comforting presence beside you. Your compassionate friend has something to tell you. It is just what you need to hear right now in your life. Listen carefully to what they have to say. Absorb every word. If no words come, that's OK too, just share in their loving company. Their presence alone is showing you that everything is going to be OK. That is enough as it is. Just be with your compassionate friend, listening out for anything you may need to hear.

Soon your friend will be getting up to leave, but before they do, they turn to you and tell you that you can call on their compassionate presence at any time. As they get up to leave, thank them for providing you with kindness and compassion when you need it most, and then bid them farewell. You are now alone again in your favourite place. Let yourself savour what just happened, reflecting on the words your compassionate friend gave to you. Know that whenever you need to, you can invite this compassionate friend to sit down beside you.

Slowly begin to bring your attention back to the feeling of your body on your seat. To your breath gently moving the body up and down. Take one last deep inhale, and on the exhale, gently open your eyes, bringing your attention back into the room.

*

Whenever you are feeling in need of some self-compassion, pop your headphones in your ears and listen to this meditation. If you are new to meditating, don't worry — this is for everyone, even if you are a beginner. If you notice your mind wandering or you find it hard to focus, this is completely normal. When this happens, simply come back to my voice and the feeling of the breath in the body to anchor you once more into the present. Repeat as required until you can effectively do this for yourself.

Examining Your Food Beliefs

Now that we've taken a look at the inner critic, we need to start examining the food beliefs that uphold the inner critic's voice. Your beliefs lead to your thoughts, which lead to your feelings, which dictate your behaviour. Therefore, to change your behaviour around food, which is the whole premise of this book, you will need to uncover and remove the faulty or problematic beliefs that maintain that behaviour through the thoughts of the inner critic and the feelings that arise as a result.

None of us are born with a plethora of food rules and beliefs, but we pick them up along the way until we end up with a perfectly formed set. Often, these food rules can be hiding in the shadows of your unconscious, but whether conscious or unconscious, they have a profound impact on your behaviours around food. These rules make it very difficult to give yourself full, unconditional permission to eat all foods, since they provide fuel for the inner critic to shout out negative barbs and statements. Your beliefs are the feeding ground for your thoughts, feelings, and behaviours, so in order to change the thoughts that arise from the inner critic, the food beliefs that maintain them need to be uncovered and challenged. Your beliefs about food are simply thoughts you have had over and over again. These thoughts originate from the food beliefs you have developed after being exposed to them through family, friends, education, mainstream media, and social media, to name a few. Some of our food beliefs may in fact be untrue and not grounded in scientific evidence, but if we lack a filter to put them through to test the truth of them, they can grow from a seed into a fully-fledged idea, taking up valuable mental space. Here are some food beliefs that I have heard over the years in clinic:

- ☐ Sugar is toxic

- ☐ Carbohydrates make you fat

- ☐ Snacking is bad

- ☐ Processed food is unhealthy

- ☐ You shouldn't eat after 7 p.m

- ☐ You should make everything from scratch

- ☐ Emotional eating is bad

You may notice that these rules are very black and white, with little room for nuance. These food beliefs are all pseudo-science that you can find in any magazine or social media feed, but that doesn't make them true. Nutrition and health is not black and white; it doesn't work like that. One food will not make you gain weight, just like it won't make you lose weight. Embracing the grey and adding space for nuance and context is a key part of shutting down your inner food critic and neutralizing the beliefs that uphold it.

Food Belief	Challenging This Belief
Sugar is toxic	All foods have a place in a healthy diet and relationship with food.
Carbohydrates make you fat	No one food makes you fat. Carbohydrates are an important source of energy and can be included in all meals and snacks.
Snacking is bad	Snacking is a way to honour your hunger and meet your needs.
Processed food is unhealthy	Many 'processed' foods are considered 'healthy', even in diet-culture land. Just because a food is processed doesn't automatically make it 'unhealthy'.
You shouldn't eat after 7 p.m	This is a rigid rule that doesn't allow for the ebb and flow of life. It's important to eat when you are hungry, no matter what time it is.
You should make everything from scratch	Making everything from scratch is not always practical or realistic. It's perfectly OK to include pre-prepared foods in your diet.
Emotional eating is bad	Emotional eating is not inherently bad. It only becomes problematic if food is your only coping mechanism,

Here are some questions you can ask yourself to challenge your own food rules and beliefs (of which there may be many):

- ☐ Where did I learn this?

- ☐ Do I know for certain that this rule or belief is grounded in evidence?

- ☐ How do I feel about this rule or belief?

- ☐ What happens when I abide by this rule or belief?

- ☐ Do I feel like it helps me or hinders me?

Eradicating Food Guilt

Food guilt doesn't have a place in a healthy relationship with food. Guilt implies that you have done something wrong. It's an emotion that arises in response to breaking a rule or moral code. Guilt and shame are sometimes used interchangeably, but they are in fact different. Guilt implies a negative evaluation of behaviour — 'I did something wrong'; whereas shame is deeper — 'I am wrong'. All emotions have a purpose, and guilt shows us when we haven't acted in alignment with our values. It's a sign that we need to redeem ourselves in some way to get back to living in alignment with these values. However, it is misguided when it arises in response to faulty and disordered beliefs about food. Eating food is not wrong, no matter what that food is. To eradicate food guilt, you must first uncover your food rules or beliefs. These beliefs are often shrouded in shoulds, musts, and have-tos and stink of diet mentality. They embody the characteristics spoken

132

about in chapter one. Here are some questions you can ask yourself to help with food guilt:

- [ ] Where did I learn that this food was bad?

- [ ] Is this true?

- [ ] What food rule have I broken that resulted in these feelings of guilt?

- [ ] Is this food rule helping or hindering me?

If you uncover sneaky food rules that are hindering your progress and eliciting food guilt after asking yourself these questions, I encourage you to go ahead and break the rule. See what happens. These rules are most likely the result of a diet culture hangover and breaking them will help to eradicate food guilt from your psyche.

Affirmations

I offer myself unconditional love, respect, and compassion.

I surrender the need for control.

I am enough; I have always been enough.

I release feelings of guilt and shame around food.

I am embracing food neutrality.

I offer myself compassion during times of suffering.

PART 2: RECONNECT

Reconnect with the needs of your mind and body to give you the information required to begin nourishing yourself with ease.

Chapter 5:

Reconnecting with the Self

'But, Niamh, I don't know what I need. Can't you just tell me?'

Most people come to me feeling lost and completely disconnected from themselves and their internal cues. They know what they 'should' do, but they just can't seem to do it. The answers cannot be found in another diet plan. It's human nature to reach for a plan or set of rules when we feel lost and don't know how to get to where we want to go. We can struggle when we don't receive a set of steps, but always having someone else tell you where to go means you never gain the skills necessary to stand on your own two feet. This part of the book is all about reconnecting you with the person who can give you all the answers – you! You'll be relieved to hear that there is a set of principles to help you do this, and I can help, but I am just your tour guide. You are the only one who can truly know what you feel and need at any given moment. I am the expert on the process, but I'm not the expert on you.

A large part of food freedom and rediscovering what health and well-being looks like for you hinges on reconnecting with your inner wisdom. This is a skill that needs to be honed, and the more you practise reconnecting with it, the stronger and easier it will become to receive its messages. Diet culture has interrupted this connection through all of its rules and regulations. The messages from diet culture are often so loud in people's minds that they drown out the sound of the voice within. Trying to reconnect with your inner wisdom while still being entrenched in diet culture is a little like trying to have a conversation with someone while listening to loud music and wearing noise-cancelling headphones. As long as you prioritize listening to loud music (diet culture), it's highly unlikely you'll be able to hear what your friend (your inner wisdom) is trying to say. The voice of your inner wisdom has not disappeared overnight, so it's unlikely that it will return overnight. It takes practice, commitment, and consistency but it's crucial to the process.

Your Inner Expert

Let me introduce you to your inner expert. Your inner expert is a wise guide that knows what you need at any given moment. Your needs will vary from day to day. It's possible to honour how you feel in the moment while keeping your future self in mind. The noise from diet culture can get so loud that it drowns out the voice of the inner expert. There is no space for it to be heard. This is why you need first to remove what you have learnt from the external world that has proven unhelpful and holds you back from truly embracing health and happiness. The key to discovering what you need can be found by tuning in to the inner expert and the wisdom it holds. Diet culture has disconnected you from this part of yourself. It's as if the phone line to the inner expert has been cut, and until it is reconnected, you cannot pick up the phone to ask yourself, 'How do I feel and what do I need?'

There is a whole weather system inside of you that requires attention. This part of the book is not about giving you more information about food and nutrition, although this has an important role in health improvement once you can unhook it from diet culture. Instead, it's about helping you reconnect with your own inner expert so that you can access your very own guide that will help you determine what and how much you need when you need it. Even if you are in the lucky minority of those who don't struggle with an eating disorder or disordered eating, connecting with the expert within will help you determine your own needs and work on your health in a way that suits you and brings you joy. If you're human, you will benefit from connecting to your inner wisdom.

Checking in with your inner expert is a little like consulting Google Maps. Making choices without consulting the map is like flying blind – how will you know the right turn to make? Reconnecting with the inner expert will help you to connect to your psychological and physiological needs. Over the years, many people have become disconnected from their internal cues and started relying on external ones like calorie counting, eating schedules, 'shoulds', and 'have-tos' to guide their food choices. Diet culture is mainly to blame for this, since it prioritizes external cues over internal ones, which is why uncovering and removing it is the premise of the first part of this book.

External cues are unreliable and not attuned to your body's unique needs. To feel grounded and at peace with food, we must prioritize messages from within.

This concept of the inner expert is based on interoception, the hidden sense we all have that holds the secret to health and well-being. If you closed your eyes now and tried to sense your heartbeat, without using your hands to find it in the body, could you locate it? This is what is meant by interoceptive awareness. Interoception is defined by Khalsa et. al in a 2018 study as 'the process by which the nervous system senses, interprets, and integrates signals originating from within the body, providing a moment-by-moment mapping of the body's internal landscape across conscious and unconscious levels'.[1] As I said, this cannot be found outside yourself. It's not found in a diet plan, an expert healthcare professional, or anyone else you look up to regarding health and wellness. It's found inside, and nobody but you can access it. Isn't that empowering? That you hold the key to everything you need? As explained by Evelyn Tribole and Elyse Resch:

interoceptive awareness is the ability to perceive physical sensations that arise from within your body. It's a direct experience, a felt sense that happens in the present moment — it's not the past or future, it happens right now. It includes basic states like feeling a distended bladder, hunger and satiety cues, and the felt sense of every emotional feeling. Every emotion has a unique physical sensation in the body. When you perceive bodily sensations, it gives rise to powerful information to help get your psychological and biological needs met.[2]

To be connected to your interoceptive awareness is to be innately connected to yourself. Not only can it support you on your journey towards food freedom, but it can also help your overall mental and emotional health, not to mention your relationships with others, whether at home, at work, or in your social circle. But how do you reconnect with it? This is where mindfulness comes in.

Mindfulness: The Key to Interoception

Mindfulness is the key to tuning in to your inner expert. Connecting to your needs through mindfulness is the first step to changing unwanted patterns and behaviours in your life, not just with food but with many other things too. Mindfulness helps us become aware of our thoughts, feelings, and behaviours at any given moment while cultivating a sense of non-judgemental acceptance. Rather than being a passive passenger in your life, you can take the wheel and become more present through formal or informal mindfulness. Formal mindfulness is practised through meditation, whereas informal mindfulness can be practised in your everyday life as you interact with the world.

It doesn't have to be complicated; we can simply think of it as becoming aware. This could look like becoming aware of your internal experiences, such as your thoughts, feelings, and bodily states, or becoming aware of the external, such as the colour of the sky, the feeling of water on your skin, or the smell of freshly cut grass in the summer. That's all it is. Presence. Rediscovering your intuitive eater and obtaining authentic health (more on this in Part 3) hinges heavily on this sense of presence and connection to the self. Without it, we can feel as if we are lost at sea without an oar. You see, your needs will change on a daily basis and no diet plan out there can know what those changes are. For example, you may feel more or less hungry some days than others, your food likes and dislikes might change, or you might need that bowl of ice cream for comfort. Diet culture doesn't allow for any of these variables.

To help my clients connect to their inner expert, I have developed an inner expert meditation that I use with them in clinic. This meditation will help you to use mindfulness to get in touch with the messages from within. You will find a script of this below, and you can download an audio version to listen to from my website nutritionwithniamh.com. I recommend listening to this a few times to help you reconnect with your own inner expert. It's normal to find this challenging, especially at the beginning, so if you struggle to remain present or gain insight into what's going on for you on the inside, don't give up. This will only come with time and practice. I promise that the more you practise this, the louder the voice of your inner expert will become, giving you access to your thoughts, feelings, bodily states, and sensations. Making time for meditation and mindfulness in your day will go a long way in helping you to reconnect with the self and fine-tune your interoceptive awareness, allowing you to become the expert of your own body.

Inner expert meditation
Let's begin by coming into a comfortable seated position. Push your back up against the back of your chair and root your feet down into the ground. If you feel comfortable, close your

eyes, or if that feels very uncomfortable, soften your gaze and look down towards the ground. Take a very slow, deep breath. Feel your sitting bones touching your seat. Move around to firmly nestle them down into the chair, giving you a greater sense of feeling grounded. Relax your face, your eyes, and in between your eyebrows. Now start to bring your attention to your breath, feeling the natural movements in your body from the movement of your breath. Notice the quality of your breathing. Is it fast or slow? Deep or shallow? Notice where your breath rests in the body. Is it high up in the chest? Is it in the midsection around your tummy or down low in the belly? Observe with curiosity instead of judgement. Continue breathing deeply and feel the cool air come in through your nose and flow all the way down to your belly. Feel your belly expand as you breathe in deeply. Feel the belly contract as you breathe out. Notice how the breath feels as it softly flows in through your nose, into your throat, and further and further down into the belly. Make sure your belly is moving slowly up and down as you inhale and exhale. Deep breaths in and out through the nose.

In your head, scan your body starting from your head and moving down towards your toes . . . How would you describe the physical sensations in your body in this moment? . . . Pleasant? . . . Unpleasant? . . . Or neutral? . . . There's no right or wrong answer here — you're just checking in with yourself.

Just notice the description that best describes how you physically feel, right now . . . Pleasant? . . . Unpleasant? . . . Or neutral? . . .

Now, take your awareness to your toes. Notice the sensations in each toe — are they warm or cold; can you feel them in your shoes? Spend a few moments there and then move your awareness upwards, into the sole of your foot, then continue upwards through the body, through the top of the foot, ankles, and lower legs, the knees and thighs. Spend a few moments in each area – be aware of all the sensations: tightness, relaxation, heat, cold, tension, aching. As you move your awareness up through your whole body, breathe into any area where you experience pain or discomfort, and then move on.

Simply observe the sensations without trying to change anything. If your mind starts to wander, bring your attention back to the breath. Now, let's start checking in with your bodily states. Are you warm, cold, or neutral? How does your bladder feel? Are you hungry? If yes, are you subtly hungry or is your hunger quite strong? Would a snack suffice, or will you soon need a meal?

Are you experiencing any emotions in this moment? Happiness, sadness, frustration, stress, tiredness? Allow everything space. Are there any physical sensations that accompany that emotion? If your mind begins to tell you a story or drag you into a narrative about the emotion, just observe it without judgement and bring your attention back to the breath. The inhale and the exhale. The rise and fall of the chest. If no emotions are present, then return your awareness to your breath, sitting peacefully and quietly. Maybe you notice a feeling of contentment – observe that too. The more you practise, the more you'll start to become aware of some of the more subtle and quieter emotions, like contentment or peace. Notice how these two also come and go. If you are struggling to feel or sit with any emotions you are experiencing, it might help to think of emotions like waves. The sea is always moving: sometimes the waves are big and strong; sometimes they're gentle and smooth. The wave always comes in, and then it always goes away. Our emotions are messengers that motivate, educate, or illuminate. If one is arising for you now:

Ask it, 'What do you want?' Listen to what it has to say.

Ask it, 'What do you need?' Listen to what it has to say.

Ask it, 'What action are you asking me to take in my life?' Listen to what it has to say.

Take a few moments to reflect on what you're experiencing in your body and mind.

If your body could speak to you now, what would it say? Is there anything it needs from you in this moment? Is there anything coming up for you right now that may need some attention later? This might be in the physical, mental, or emotional body. If the inner expert had a voice, what would it say to you now?

Now, slowly bring your attention back to your breath. Feel the movement of the breath in the body. Slowly bring your hands together and rub your palms together to generate some heat. Gently place them over your eyes. Take one last deep inhale and blink open your eyes into your hands, readjusting to the light in the room. Slowly lower your hands from your face in your own time, bringing your awareness back into the room. Well done. You've just practised the inner expert meditation. The more you practise this, the more attuned you will become to the messages from within.

*

Mindfulness will help you to listen to the whispers from within the body so that it doesn't have to shout so loud to be heard. The more attuned and aware you are, the better you will be at attending to the needs of the mind and body and, therefore, the more able you will be to treat it with the loving care it deserves.

Affirmations

I trust my inner expert.

I am becoming more connected to myself every day.

I listen to the whispers within.

I create space in my life to connect to myself.

My body knows best.

I am wise beyond belief.

Chapter 6:

Reconnecting with Hunger

Ah, hunger. The enemy when you're trying to diet or lose weight. We've all been there and experienced that dreaded feeling when you're still hours away from your allocated meal-time — or you've gone to bed early so as not to feel those hunger pangs. Some clients say they see hunger as a sign that weight loss is happening. Red flags — hello! Is it any wonder that dieting is one of the biggest predictors of developing an eating disorder? Hunger is a sign that your body is working as it should, but diet culture teaches you that it's something to be beaten and conquered. You will never win the fight against hunger — hunger will always win out because food is the only effective appetite suppressant. Nothing else will do. Here are some things diet culture will tell you to try in order to suppress hunger:

☐ You're probably just thirsty. Have a glass of water instead.

☐ Drink a glass of water before a meal to reduce the amount of food you eat.

☐ Fill up on salad before you eat any carbohydrates.

☐ Just have some popcorn/fruit/other low-calorie snack.

☐ Why not take up smoking?

OK, so maybe the last one is a bit of an exaggeration, but these are things people have told me they tried to lose weight or maintain their weight loss. To be clear, none of these strategies are healthy or kind to the body since they require you to deny the body what it needs. Depriving the body of what it needs will only work temporarily; eventually, those needs catch up with you. Here are some of the things that can happen when you don't honour your hunger cues by eating something or eating enough food when you do:

☐ Overeating

☐ Binge eating

☐ Emotional overeating

☐ Feeling out of control around food

☐ Having an insatiable appetite when you eventually do eat something

☐ Feeling a lack of satisfaction

☐ Obsessing about food

I could go on. Learning to reconnect with your hunger cues and eating in response to them is integral to resolving all of the above. It is the first bodily signal to try to connect with, as it underpins the rest; if your hunger needs are not met, it will be very difficult to hear and honour your other cues, such as fullness and satisfaction.

The Four Types of Hunger

Many of my clients are surprised to hear that there are different types of hunger. There is a myth that intuitive eating means 'to eat when you're hungry and stop when you're full'. It's not quite this simple – to me, this sounds like just another rule. Remember, a diet is anything that restricts what, when, or how much you eat. Well, that sure sounds like a diet, right? If you were to tell me that I could only eat when I was physically hungry, I would instantly feel anxious about all the situations in the future where I would have to control myself and say no to food when I really wanted to say yes:

- ☐ That cake at a friend's birthday.

- ☐ A bar of chocolate with a cup of tea in front of Netflix.

- ☐ Sharing a dessert with a partner at dinner.

- ☐ Trying out some street food on holidays.

- ☐ Eating popcorn at the cinema.

These are all experiences I would potentially miss out on because of the 'only eat when hungry' rule. We don't only eat as a response to physical hunger. That sounds pretty boring to me. Food is so much more than fuel. It provides us with joy, pleasure, connection, and comfort. Reducing food to fuel by placing a rule on ourselves that 'we must be physically hungry to eat' has the potential to remove all the joy from the eating experience. We eat for many different reasons, and most of these can be grouped into the following four categories:

1. Physical hunger — eating in response to physical hunger cues

2. Taste hunger — eating something for pure pleasure, even if you're not physically hungry

3. Practical hunger — eating in the absence of physical hunger cues to look after your future self

4. Emotional hunger — eating in response to an emotion

These four types of hunger are all normal parts of being human. Diet culture has made people believe that there's something wrong with them or they're doing something terrible if they decide to enjoy ice cream when they're not hungry or eat some cake at a birthday party. In reality, this is what I would call a normal and healthy relationship with food. Knowing that it's perfectly acceptable to eat in the absence of hunger cues is often very liberating for the people I have worked with. This doesn't mean that you eat without consulting your hunger, fullness, and satisfaction cues. A connection to these cues is integral to making choices that satisfy you and make your body feel well. Just because you *can* eat, doesn't mean you always should or that it is the right solution to the need at hand. This chapter will teach you how to consult your hunger cues so that you can choose accordingly.

The Importance of Honouring Hunger

It was 2017. At the time, I worked an office job and tried to attend a yoga class after work a few times a week. It was often the highlight of my day – and still is! There was usually a large block of time between my lunch and an evening class, so I would try to top up my energy stores by having a snack before the class. On this particular day, for some reason, that didn't happen – probably because I wasn't prepared or was too busy at work and forgot. I remember specifically that on the week in question I had a lot on my mind. I find that when I am mentally preoccupied, I am less connected to my body and its cues. I felt absolutely fine when I walked into the class and rolled out my yoga mat – I didn't feel hungry, nor was I aware of any subtle hunger cues. But by the time I came into my first downward-facing dog, my blood sugar plummeted and I started to sweat and shake – a sure sign that I needed food, and fast. I was suddenly so hungry that there was no option other than to roll up my mat and leave the class. Luckily, like a true nutritionist, I always have emergency food reserves in my car – but this time, that only extended to a packet of oatcakes. Now, I don't know if you've ever eaten dry oatcakes, but I wouldn't say it's the most satisfying experience. Those oatcakes were eaten in five minutes flat — a new record! I couldn't get them into me quick enough. Fifteen minutes later, the shakes still hadn't left me. I can almost guarantee you that if there had been a Mars bar or a bottle of Coke in the car, I would have chosen either of those over the oatcakes — nutrition degree or not. Let me explain why.

When you experience a feeling of intense hunger, aka primal hunger, all logic leaves the room. This is not a time when you access nutrition information or give yourself the chance to ask what it is you would truly like to eat. The body takes over and your physiological need for food will win out. No amount of intellect, knowledge, or willpower will override this process. It is akin to holding your breath underwater. No matter how much you tell yourself that you'll take a gentle, slow, and elegant inhale when you come to the surface, the longer you deprive the body of air, the more gasping the inhalation of breath will be when you gain access to it. It's the exact same with food. It's a survival instinct.

When you reach a stage of primal hunger, the production of two main hormones that trigger this physiological drive to eat is accelerated: ghrelin and neuropeptide Y (NPY). Ghrelin is released in response to hunger, to get you to eat. Neuropeptide Y is what I like to call the 'carb fairy' hormone. This is the hormone that drives the urge to consume carbo-hydrates when you feel especially hungry. You know that feeling of wanting pasta, pizza, bread, and cake when you're dieting? Chances are that NPY is driving that process, and how amazing is it that you have this inbuilt mechanism to ensure you get the nutrition that you need? Carbohydrate is the body and brain's preferred source of energy. Without it, your physiological needs will not be fulfilled and you will feel hungry. A lot.

Hunger is not something to be feared. You can trust that if your body is giving you a hunger signal, you can honour it by eating something. My clients have asked me if they should honour every hunger cue, even if they are experiencing hunger a lot. Yes, you absolutely should. Doing this is treating yourself with kindness and respect by providing nourishment when your body tells you that it needs it. We know that dieting can result in increased hunger signals – for example, ghrelin levels can remain elevated for up to two years after a period of restriction. Honouring every hunger cue will rebuild trust between you and your body, reassuring the body that food is freely available. The more you do this, the more the body will trust that you will feed it adequately when it needs nourishment. If you don't do this, the body will remain on high alert, waiting for the next famine period. Essentially, you need to reassure the body that you have its back. Until then, the body will continue to look after itself by doing all it can to make you eat.

Reconnecting with Your Hunger Cues

For a lot of my clients, learning to honour their hunger is a transformative development in rebuilding their relationship with food. They are often amazed at the power it can hold. Some people reconnect with their hunger cues in a matter of weeks; other people can take a couple of months to rediscover them. Whatever pace you move at is exactly where you need to be. When you start trying to reconnect with these cues, you may find it challenging at first if your subtle hunger cues are deeply buried within. You may have been denying them for a long time, and if so, it can take a while for them to resurface. This is normal. Think of it like this: every time you have followed a diet rule rather than honouring your hunger cues, you buried your hunger cues a little deeper under the surface. The deeper they are buried, the longer it may take to get to them.

When you begin to reconnect with your hunger cues, I recommend you ensure a regular eating pattern – about every three to four hours. This is not a rule, hence why I am not advising you on what or how much to eat – that's for you to decide based on your internal cues of hunger, fullness, and satisfaction. I also don't want you to beat yourself up if you don't manage to do this all the time. Life is messy and it's not possible to have a perfect pattern of eating. There will be days when you don't eat for hours, forget to eat, or don't plan in advance and end up eating something that doesn't make you feel well. I'm a nutritionist and have a very healthy relationship with food and this still happens to me from time to time. Remember the perfectionistic and all-or-nothing thinking we spoke about in Chapter 4? We don't want that to resurface here. Eating regularly will ensure you are adequately nourished and help to kick-start your hunger cues. It gives you a flexible guideline to follow when you are in the early stages of rediscovering your intuitive eater, which can be very helpful. Flexible guidelines are helpful, but rigid rules are not.

The hunger fullness scale, as originally developed by Evelyn Tribole and Elyse Resch, is the best learning tool to help you begin reconnecting with these cues.[1] The scale ranges from zero to ten and will help you reconnect with the subtle cues of hunger, which is an important part of predicting your future food needs. When I show this to people in clinic, they usually recognize the over-hungry and the overfull stages but find it difficult to connect with how the middle category, the normal eating range, feels in their own body. This makes sense, given how diet culture encourages us to disconnect from these cues and eat the bare minimum as part of the quest to control weight.

When you start eating from a stage of primal hunger, a zero or one on the scale, chances are you'll eat that meal or snack in record time. It takes about twenty minutes for the body to register fullness; if you are eating from a stage of primal hunger, I can almost guarantee you will finish before this. We've all been there – feeling so hungry that we've finished a meal in five minutes; hence that saying of 'inhaling your food'. You miss the finish line when you eat food quickly, since there is no space or time to tune in to the subtle cues of fullness. If you only eat when you feel extremely hungry, you will overeat. You might even feel out of control around food. But overeating is a normal response to primal hunger. It doesn't mean you are out of control or addicted to food. I can't tell you how many times certain food issues, such as overeating and bingeing, have resolved for the people I have worked with once they begin to honour their hunger cues. It is an integral part of recovery.

As a guideline, it's best to eat when experiencing a hunger level of two, three, or four and to stop eating when feeling a fullness level of six or seven on the scale. Again, this is a guideline, not a rule. It's not always this straightforward. For example, you might have a busy day and your last chance to eat arrives when you are at a five on the scale (practical hunger). Likewise, you might be out for dinner and the food is so good that you overeat to an eight or a nine (taste hunger). As long as it isn't all of the time, there is absolutely nothing wrong with this. It probably wouldn't feel very good in your body to eat like this all of the time, but it feels great to have the freedom and choice to do so when you need to or just want to. That's what true food freedom feels like.

The Hunger Fullness Scale

	Rating	Description of hunger fullness sensation
Over-hungry	0	Primal hunger, feels very intense and urgent
Over-hungry	1	Hangry, anxious to eat
Over-hungry	2	Very hungry, looking forward to eating
Normal eating range	3	Hungry and ready to eat but without urgency, polite hunger
Normal eating range	4	Subtly hungry, slightly empty
Normal eating range	5	Neutral — neither hungry nor full
Normal eating range	6	Beginning to feel emerging fullness

Normal eating range	7	Comfortable fullness, satisfied and content
Overfull	8	A little too full, just tipped over the edge
Overfull	9	Very full or too full, Christmas-dinner feeling
Overfull	10	Painfully full, stuffed, feelings of nausea

The Hunger Sensations

Hunger is present long before it grows into the obvious signs of a stomach ache and gnawing in the belly. If you are only attuned to the signs of primal hunger, it will be very difficult to attend to your needs in time. The subtle signs of hunger can show up in many ways. It is these subtle signs that you need to look out for. They can show up in five different areas of the physical, emotional, and mental body: body, stomach, head, mood, and energy. All of the hunger sensations, both subtle and obvious, are included in the list below:

☐ Body — shaking, quivering, sweating, salivating at the thought of food

☐ Stomach — emptiness, gnawing, stomach ache, gurgling, rumbling, hunger pangs

☐ Head — poor concentration, lack of focus, distracted, thinking about food, dizzy, light-headed, achiness

☐ Mood — hangry, irritable, cranky, snappy, moody, restless

☐ Energy — sleepy, fatigued, unproductive, sluggish

This list is not exhaustive, and once you begin reconnecting with your hunger cues, you may find that you have your own quirks or telltale signs that hunger is upon you. For example, when I hit a one on the hunger scale, I find myself crouching in front of the corner press. I only ever do this when I'm getting close to primal hunger and it's a sure sign I need a meal very soon. When I find myself at a three or four on the scale, I start to lose focus and concentration — which means it's essential that I am well fuelled before heading into any of my client sessions. My friends also say that I get very quiet when I'm hungry and tend to respond to them with one-word answers. One of my clients sneezes when she's starting to feel hungry! These are all subtle signs of hunger. Nothing is off the table — no matter how weird. Only you will understand what hunger feels like in your body.

The hunger scan is a meditation you can use to help you get in touch with your hunger cues. You can download the audio version from my website. I suggest listening to this a number of times — just once isn't going to cut the mustard. Practice makes progress, so the more you do this, the easier it will become to get in touch with your hunger signals and the faster you will get at it. Eventually, once you get to know yourself and your hunger cues, you will be able to scan the body in a few seconds and determine where you lie on the hunger fullness scale.

The Hunger Scan (Adapted from Evelyn Tribole)
Get yourself nice and comfortable. Take a few deep breaths in through your nose, and out through your mouth. In through your nose, and out through your mouth. And once more, in through your nose and out through your mouth. And then gently close your eyes . . .

Let's start by getting in touch with your physical body. Relax your face, your eyes and between your eyebrows. Take a few moments to settle your body. In your head, scan your body, starting from your head and moving down towards your toes . . .

How would you describe the physical sensations in your body in this moment? Pleasant? Unpleasant? Or neutral? There's no right or wrong answer here – you're just checking in with yourself.

Just notice the description that best describes how you phys-ically feel, right now. Pleasant? Unpleasant? Or neutral? . . .

Now we're going to look at some key areas where hunger can show up in the body, starting with the more subtle and nuanced signs of hunger . . .

I'd like you to begin by bringing your attention to your mood. Sometimes biological hunger is experienced by a shift in mood. You may feel irritable or cranky. Notice your mood right now in this moment. Do you feel a little snappy or curt? Do you feel a little low? . . .

If so, these may be signs that you're beginning to experience hunger. Just take notice, without judgement . . .

Now I'd like you to shift your attention to your overall energy level. Sometimes biological hunger is experienced by a dip in energy, characterized by fatigue or even sleepiness. Do you feel sluggish and tired and it has nothing to do with a bad night's sleep? Or maybe you feel unusually blah or a bit listless? . . .

Again, just notice if you experience these initial signs of hunger by a shift in your energy . . .

Now I'd like you to shift your attention to the more easily detectable hunger signals, starting with your head, so just bring your awareness to your head . . .

Sometimes biological hunger is experienced as a physical sensation in your head, so just notice any physical sensations in your head right now. How would you describe the way it feels to you? . . .

Is there a slight ache? Are you light-headed, or does it feel like you're zoning out? Maybe you feel a little dizzy or even a bit faint? Are you having any difficulty concentrating? Whatever the sensation, just notice . . .

If you're experiencing any of these sensations, it's possible that you're experiencing a degree of hunger . . .

Just notice it without judgement.

Now, move your attention to your stomach.

What would best describe the physical sensation in your stomach right now? . . .

Would you describe it as a gentle rumbling or gurgling? Or maybe it feels empty? . . . Or maybe there's an uncomfortable pain, a stomach ache . . .

Are there any hunger pangs or a gnawing feeling in your belly? Or does your stomach feel comfortable or neutral? . . .

What is the physical sensation in your stomach? Be aware that any of these sensations may be signalling hunger . . .

Perhaps you're experiencing other physical sensations that might be indicating you're hungry. Maybe you find yourself salivating at the thought of food and of eating. Or maybe you feel kind of shaky and like you have low blood sugar, another physical symptom of hunger indicating you need to eat . . .

Now I'd like you to take a brief scan of all of these elements, starting from your mood . . .

Now your energy level . . .

Now your physical sensations, in your head and your stomach and anywhere else you might be experiencing them . . .

Now I'd like you to consider all of these elements together, and with that overall consideration, I'd like you to rate your hunger level on a hunger/fullness scale from zero to ten. Ten is so full you feel sick, and it's painful . . .

Zero is painfully empty, and five is completely neutral, neither empty nor full. So how would you rate your hunger right now? . . .

Keep in mind, whatever number you rate, it's not right or wrong. It's just a process to help you get in touch, and the more you get familiar with the sensations, the easier it will become to tell when you're hungry.

Good. Now I'd like you to take a few deep breaths in through your nose, and out through your mouth. In through your nose, and out through your mouth. And once more, in through your nose, and out through your mouth. Open your eyes, and bring your attention back into the room.

Bridging the Gap

Let me introduce you to a little strategy I like to call 'bridging the gap'. This one very simple strategy is going to save you from the dreaded primal hunger I've explained above. Are you ready? Here it is: plan ahead. Primal hunger will happen sometimes. And because we know what it causes, it's best to try and prevent it as much as possible. Bridging the gap will help you avoid going long periods of time without eating, but to do this, you will need to plan ahead. This could look like:

- Having snacks ready to go in places you often frequent e.g. the car, office or anywhere else you spend a lot of your time.

- Batch cooking meals and having them ready to go in the fridge or freezer when you're short on time.

- Looking at your schedule ahead of time and roughly planning when you will have time to take a break to eat.

- Snacking on something to 'bridge the gap' between mealtimes.

This strategy is a form of looking after your future self. You will thank your past self for planning ahead when you find yourself in sticky situations with no quick access to food. When I speak to people who have young children and relate it to caring for those children, they instantly get it. Any parent that I know would rarely leave the house with their children without packing snacks — just in case. Although it may look different for you as an adult, the purpose is the same: to avoid going long periods of time without eating. If you pair reconnecting with your hunger cues with practical strategies that prevent primal hunger and therefore nourish your body adequately, you will soon begin to reap the rewards.

Affirmations

Hunger is a friend, not an enemy.

It is safe for me to listen to my body's hunger cues.

I honour every hunger cue by eating something.

I give my body the sustenance it requires.

My body deserves to be fed.

It is safe for me to eat.

Chapter 7:

Reconnecting with Satisfaction

Do you know what you love to eat? If yes, do you allow yourself to enjoy those foods without guilt? Deriving pleasure from food is a critical part of having a healthy relationship with it. If you're not satisfied, you're not happy. It's as simple as that. Diet culture has removed pleasure as an important component of the eating experience. We have been conditioned to believe that 'food is fuel' and that enjoying your food too much is hedonistic and greedy. What utter diet culture BS! Satisfaction is a core goal in intuitive eating, and rediscovering pleasure and enjoyment in food will mean you are much less likely to reach for food outside of mealtimes. Let me tell you a story to demonstrate.

Ruth is considering what to have for her dinner this evening. She thinks she would like a warming chicken curry but then remembers she heard somewhere that coconut milk is bad for you. She knows that a chicken salad is considered 'good for you', so she decides to have that instead.

After dinner, while watching TV, she starts thinking about the chocolate and crisps in the press . . . 'No, I've done well all day. I shouldn't,' she tells herself. She grabs an apple instead.

Still not satisfied thirty minutes later, she grabs a banana, a yoghurt, and some jellies her kids brought home from school.

Still not satisfied, and feeling frustrated from eating some jellies, she says, 'Screw it,' opens the press, grabs the chocolate, eats it, and goes to bed feeling uncomfortably full. 'Tomorrow is a new day,' she tells herself.

Can you identify with any part of Ruth's story? When I tell this story in my group coaching programme, people usually respond with little titters of laughter because they can see themselves in Ruth. They've been there, often many times over. This is what happens when we don't listen to our satisfaction cues. The desire doesn't go away: the cravings only get stronger, and you end up eating much more than you would have if you had just given yourself what you wanted in the first place. Eating a salad when you really want a curry will not lead to satisfaction and will only encourage overeating later on. The best way to rid yourself of a craving is to eat the food you're craving. Have you ever tried eating the 'good' version of a food, only to be left wanting afterwards? Reconnecting with your satisfaction cues and honouring them is your next step on the intuitive eating path that will help you determine what and how much food you need to feel satisfied. It will remove the confusion around what to eat and what not to eat, as the body will always give you this information readily — once you know how to tune into it.

Fullness vs Satisfaction

So what do I mean when I use the word satisfaction and how does it relate to fullness? Fullness is the physical sensation of satiety. Satisfaction is the mental sensation of satiety — that feeling of being wholly and completely satisfied with the food or meal you've eaten. If a meal contains a certain amount of energy, it will provide fullness, but that doesn't mean it will provide satisfaction. For example, let's take two different meals and say that they each provide 1000 kcals:

1. Ribeye steak and gravy

2. Steak, roast potatoes, roast vegetables, and gravy

What meal do you think would be more satisfying? Technically, since both of these meals contain the same amount of energy, they would each provide fullness, but I'm guessing you would feel more satisfied after meal two. As humans, we are hard-wired to seek satisfaction from food, and without achieving this, the drive to eat will remain. A lack of satisfaction only encourages overeating and bingeing later on. Likewise, it's possible for some foods to provide satisfaction but not fullness, such as chocolate, crisps, and other desserts. These foods may lead to taste satisfaction, but not body satisfaction.

Taste and Body Satisfaction

When I speak about satisfaction, I'm referring to not just the pleasure you derive from food, but also to how food feels in the body. This is something that people often miss on their intuitive eating journey. Yes, it's incredibly important for food to taste good and to reach taste satisfaction, but not always at the expense of body satisfaction. Your body will give you signs about what foods feel good and what foods do not feel good. Continuing to eat food that satisfies taste hunger but does not satisfy the body is not true intuitive eating and will most likely lead to you feeling unwell in your body.

As explained earlier, at the beginning of your intuitive eating journey, you will most likely be eating food that does not make you feel well, perhaps even a lot of these foods, especially if they have been previously restricted. This may seem counter-intuitive but it is normal and expected. Eventually this honeymoon stage ends, and you won't crave these foods as much, as you know you can have them whenever you wish. Then, you are truly free to check in with how food feels, both from a taste and body satisfaction perspective. This helps you to make choices about food using intuitive eating skills, rather than external rules about what is deemed 'good' or 'bad'.

Questions to uncover taste satisfaction include:

- ☐ What do I feel like eating?

- ☐ Will I enjoy this food?

- ☐ What are my taste preferences?

Questions to uncover body satisfaction include:

- ☐ How hungry am I?

☐ Do I want something light, airy, heavy, filling, or in between?

☐ How will my stomach feel after finishing eating?

The Three T's

When you move away from dieting and into intuitive eating, it's normal to feel a little lost around food or struggle to answer the question 'What would I like to eat right now?' This makes sense, especially if you have relied on a diet or meal plan to guide your food choices up to this point. You are relearning how to eat from the ground up and this will take time. You're rediscovering your likes and dislikes around food. This is the fun part. You get to explore food without the confines of diet culture rules. How exciting!

I love providing my clients with quick-fire ways to check in with their needs, and in this case, you can use the three T's – taste, texture, and temperature – to discover what it is you want to eat. Whenever you're unsure what it is you'd like to eat, check in with yourself by asking:

☐ Taste: Would I like something sweet, savoury, salty, bitter, or spicy?

☐ Texture: Would I like something smooth, soft, crunchy, chewy, or a mix?

☐ Temperature: Would I like hot, cold, or room-temperature food?

The more you ask yourself these questions, the easier it will be to uncover your true food likes and dislikes — not just those that diet culture has deemed you 'should' or 'should not' like or dislike. Every time you ask yourself these questions and stay present with the eating experience, you are recording another food experience in your psyche to tap into in the future, informing you whether or not you would like to make that choice again. It's not uncommon for people to realize they don't actually enjoy foods they thought they loved as they go through the intuitive eating process. This is mainly due to these foods being taken off a pedestal. If you place some foods above others, they become forbidden fruit and remain more desirable than others. Once you embrace food neutrality, you are free to tune into your satisfaction cues and uncover whether you genuinely enjoy the food or not.

Dropping Perfection

I remember a conversation I had with a client in my practice about finding satisfaction with food. She loved the idea of giving in to her cravings and allowing herself to choose the foods she really desired. It felt very freeing and liberating to do so. But then she gave me a perfect example demonstrating the importance of embracing imperfection while finding satisfaction with food. She told me she had arrived home from work with a real craving for chicken casserole, but she didn't have the ingredients or energy to prepare it that day. Rather than throwing in the towel and deciding that she wasn't going to be satisfied with her dinner, she compromised and chose something that provided some level of satisfaction. At the same time, she made a mental note to go shopping for the ingredients for a chicken casserole the next day.

You may not always be able to satisfy your cravings for several reasons, which is why embracing imperfection and flexibility is necessary. This may happen when, for example:

- ☐ You do not have the ingredients to hand for the meal you really want.

- ☐ Your local restaurant has discontinued your favourite dish.

- ☐ You are disappointed with a meal you prepared.

- ☐ You get runny poached eggs in a café, having ordered hard.

- ☐ You get served vegetables that are mushy, instead of al dente.

Sometimes you will want something that is not currently available to you – this is normal. I don't want to set you up with unrealistic standards that do not translate into real life (ahem, diet mentality, hello!). In these moments, when the food you crave is not available, try your best to satisfy yourself with what *is* available, or make a note to buy or prepare the food you desire for next time. It's not going to be perfect all of the time.

Mindful Eating

Mindful eating is a powerful way to tune into your satisfaction cues. It will help you to connect with and explore food while bringing curiosity to the experience of eating without judgement. Applying mindfulness to food will allow you to notice how food feels in your mouth, mind, and body. Mindful eating applies all the principles of mindfulness to the eating experience — you are simply being present with food. You can do this by stepping into the senses, since they're the gateway to assessing both taste and body satisfaction.

One of my favourite exercises to do with clients to help them experience mindful eating is a chocolate meditation, which always elicits a bit of excitement! This exercise places your full sensory attention on the chocolate as you eat it and it usually results in a lot of insights. I have heard many times from people that it felt like a completely new experience — that's the power of intentional attention. Although mindful eating can sometimes result in eating less food, that shouldn't be why it's used. If your intention in practising mindful eating is to eat less, you're missing the point. This will keep you disconnected from the present — the base premise of mindfulness. My description of mindful eating I use in clinic is based on the guidelines laid out by The Center for Mindful Eating.[1] This organization is headed up by a trusted colleague and holds the same values as the non-diet approach. You are a mindful eater if you:

- ☐ Allow your hunger and fullness cues to guide your decision of when to eat and when to stop eating

- ☐ Allow your satisfaction cues to guide your food choices, while paying equal attention to how food tastes and feels in your body

☐ Approach your individual food likes and dislikes with curiosity instead of judgment

Someone who eats mindfully:

☐ Is aware of and reflects upon the effects of mind-less eating

☐ Consciously directs awareness to all aspects of the eating experience in the present moment

☐ Pays attention to the immediate effects associated with food choices and not just to the distant health outcome of that choice

☐ Acknowledges that there is no right or wrong way to eat, but that all food experiences provide us with information to guide future food choices

☐ Uses any insights collected from being present and mindful with food to achieve specific health goals

Mindful eating is a sensual experience. Your senses should be used to savour, taste and explore food. Using the five senses, you can ask yourself the below questions to apply mindfulness to the eating experience:

☐ Sight – what does the food look like? Can you notice anything specific about it? What colour is it? Does it have any designs or patterns? Is there a variety of different colours?

☐ Smell — what does the food smell like? Is it subtle or strong? Is the smell pleasant, unpleasant, or neutral?

☐ Touch — what does the food feel like in your hands or mouth? Can you notice any specific textures? How does it feel as you swallow it? What temperature is the food?

☐ Taste — what does the food taste like? Do you enjoy the taste of it?

☐ Sound — does the food make a sound when you place it in your hands or mouth?

Satisfaction Saturation

I love Häagen-Dazs salted caramel ice cream — It's my absolute favourite (I could say the same for anything that contains salted caramel). When I invest in a tub of Häagen-Dazs (if you know, you know), I really want to spend time enjoying it. Those first few spoonfuls are absolute heaven, but the taste begins to fade over time, and the tenth spoon isn't ever as good as the first. Don't get me wrong, it still tastes incredible, but it hasn't quite got the sparkle of the first few bites. Does this sound familiar, or can you relate it to the experience of eating one of your favourite foods?

This decline in flavour as exposure increases is a phenomenon scientists call sensory specific satiety. As a food or drink is consumed, the pleasantness of its sensory qualities declines, leading to what I have coined 'satisfaction saturation'. Your taste buds begin to become desensitized to the taste. When you begin eating food, you do so for several different reasons, as illustrated in the graph on the next page. No matter the reason for eating, sensory pleasure will be at its strongest in those first few bites, particularly if you are eating food you enjoy until you reach the point of peak satisfaction. Once you hit this point, if you continue eating, satisfaction will only decrease, leading to uncomfortable levels of fullness. As we have already defined, when we refer to satisfaction we are talking about both taste and body satisfaction. Using mindfulness to become aware of when satisfaction saturation occurs is a skill that will help you stop eating once you have reached this point, because why continue if your taste buds are saturated? Without being mindful, you are likely to miss the point of satisfaction saturation.

Picture yourself in the cinema, engrossed in a movie, enjoying your box of popcorn. Ever felt your fingers brushing the bottom of the box without even realizing you've eaten the whole lot? When you are distracted or eat mindlessly, it's very easy to eat until a meal or snack is gone, rather than until you reach the point of peak satisfaction. This means that you will be relying on external, rather than internal, cues to guide your eating. Mindful eating will help you to avoid this, as it encourages you to check in to the present moment and whether the food still tastes good or feels good in the body.

To help you uncover this point of satisfaction saturation, stay present with your food by using your skills of mindfulness and keep the below question in mind:

If I continue to eat this food, will my satisfaction increase or decrease?

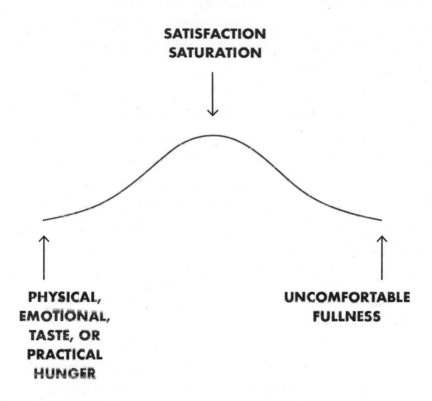

SATISFACTION SATURATION

PHYSICAL, EMOTIONAL, TASTE, OR PRACTICAL HUNGER

UNCOMFORTABLE FULLNESS

Reconnecting with Your Satisfaction Cues

Remember that chocolate meditation I mentioned earlier? Well, you're in luck because I've included it here. The transcription is below and you can download an audio version from nutritionwithniamh.com.

Chocolate meditation (adapted from Just Eat It *by Laura Thomas)* Welcome to this mindful eating meditation. This meditation will help you to get in touch with your senses and the experience of eating. You will need some wrapped chocolate to complete this practice. Once you have that, let's begin.

Get yourself nice and comfortable . . .

Take a few deep breaths, in through your nose and out through your mouth . . .

Settle into your body. Relax your face, your eyes and in between your eyebrows. Part the lips ever so slightly to allow the jaw to relax.

Now look at the chocolate in your hand; notice the shiny foil . . .

Are there any patterns or designs on the wrapper?

Gently closing your eyes, move the chocolate around in your hands. Rub your fingers over the foil and feel the textures and shape of the chocolate underneath. Can you trace any ridges or designs on the chocolate itself? Feel the weight of the chocolate, is it dense or is it light? Imagine what's inside the foil. Smooth rich chocolate that will melt when you put it in your mouth. Maybe there's caramel in the middle or maybe it has notes of orange or vanilla. Perhaps there are some nuts or crunchy pieces inside. For now just imagine what it's going to taste like as you bite into it. Is it hard or soft and melty? Is it solid or filled in the centre? . . .

Now open your eyes and gently peel back the foil. Listen to the sound of the foil crinkling as you unwrap it. Take a look at the chocolate underneath. Gaze at it as though you've never seen a chocolate like this before. What do you see? How would you describe the chocolate? Is it textured or patterned or completely smooth? What colour is it? Is it rich and dark or milky and creamy? Anticipate the flavours in your mouth. Are they smooth or are they sharp and bitter? . . .

Now lift the chocolate up to your nose and take a deep breath in. What do you smell? Just notice all the different scents of the chocolate. What does it smell like? Does it smell sweet or bitter? Can you pick out the different scents? Vanilla, cocoa, maybe butterscotch or honey, brown sugar, orange blossom or mint. Notice any sensations that you might experience in your mouth, stomach, or elsewhere in your body . . .

Now it's time to take a bite of the chocolate, but don't chew it yet. Let the flavours melt onto your tongue. What do you taste? What flavours are present? Is it the same as what you expected? What are the textures you feel? How does it feel on your tongue as you slowly roll it around your mouth? Does the flavour change over time or as you slowly begin to chew? Does it get stuck on your teeth or on the roof of your mouth? . . .

When you're ready, go ahead and swallow. Notice the sensation on the back of your tongue travelling down towards your stomach. How does it feel in your stomach and elsewhere in your body? . . .

Now take a second and a third bite. Does the chocolate change flavours? Is it as good as the first bite?

You can continue eating or you can begin to make your way out by gently taking a few deep breaths. In through your nose and out through your mouth. On the next exhale, slowly begin to blink open your eyes and bring your attention back into the room. Well done for making it through this mindful eating meditation. You can bring what you have learnt here into future experiences with food to increase your satisfaction levels.[2]

Affirmations

Every time I honour my cravings, I am rebuilding trust in my body.

It is safe for me to listen to my body's satisfaction cues.

It is safe for me to feel content and satisfied.

I joyfully observe the sensory qualities of this meal.

I appreciate and give thanks for this food.

I give myself permission to enjoy my food.

Chapter 8:

Reconnecting with Fullness

Any chance you've jumped to this chapter before reading the ones that come before it? If so, I strongly encourage you to go back and read them in sequence. When people start working with me in clinic, they often have an urgent desire to be told how to stop eating when they're full. It's one of the most common questions I am asked at the start of someone's intuitive eating journey. It might surprise you that, out of all the topics I speak about in clinic, fullness is one I spend the least amount of time teaching clients about! This is because fullness often sorts itself out, at least to a large degree, when hunger and satisfaction are understood and honoured and when you give yourself unconditional permission to eat all foods. Without first working on these principles, it will be impossible to stop eating when full. So if you have jumped forward, this is your sign to trust the process and head back to the previous chapters, knowing that they all play a role in helping you to stop eating when full. None of the topics discussed in this book work in a vacuum. They all weave together and work synergistically in some way, shape or form.

You cannot 'will' yourself to stop eating when full. This only comes with time once you have made up for the scarcity left over from dieting and rebuilt trust with your body. In order to honour your fullness, you will need to give yourself the food you desire, otherwise it will be very hard to stop eating when full. However, there are some things you can do to help, once you've implemented the steps discussed in the previous chapters.

The Fullness Sensations

What does fullness feel like in your body? Can you distinguish between comfortable and uncomfortable levels of fullness? Fullness is not simply the absence of hunger. If you stop eating just as the feelings of hunger dissipate, you will most likely find yourself hungry again soon after. This is why the optimum time to stop eating is when you reach a seven on the hunger fullness scale. It's common for people to struggle with identifying comfortable sensations of fullness. Most people can clearly recognize what it feels like to be stuffed and uncomfortable but find it difficult to identify the feeling of comfortable satiety. This may take some exploration, just like uncovering your hunger cues did; but remember, if you begin eating from primal hunger it will be very difficult, I would say nearly impossible, to notice comfortable fullness, simply because of the sheer speed at which you will eat your meal.

Just like hunger, the subtle signs of fullness can show up in different ways. There are five different areas of the physical, emotional, and mental body that they can show up in: body, stomach, head, mood, and energy.

☐ Body — not interested in food, food no longer makes you salivate, reduced cravings, eating slows down

☐ Stomach — comfortable, gently full, slightly bloated/burpy, gurgling/digesting

☐ Head — improved concentration, focused, clear

☐ Mood — calm, content, happy, satisfied, satiated

☐ Energy — recharged, energized, sleepy

The above are only guidelines. Discovering what comfortable fullness feels like in your body is unique to you and may take some time and attention to discover.

Obstacles to Feeling Your Fullness

When you begin to try and reconnect with your fullness cues, removing any obstacles that prevent you from doing so is essential. The following obstacles are the ones I come across most in clinic, and sometimes removing them is enough to begin honouring fullness cues. If you remove all of the obstacles below and still struggle with stopping eating when comfortably full, don't panic. Every person's journey looks different and moves at a different pace. Ensure you are getting enough nourishment and variety in your diet, you are honouring your hunger and satisfaction cues, and you're giving yourself full unconditional permission to eat all foods. Still, you may need to amp up your connection to your fullness cues and practise presence with meals. If you are still overeating, you may be using food to cope with your emotions; Chapter 9 is dedicated to helping you uncover and overcome this. It's not uncommon for this part of the process to take some time — don't compare yourself to anyone else. It will come.

Clean plate syndrome
Clean plate syndrome is the need to finish all of the food on your plate without consulting your hunger, fullness, or satis-faction cues. This comes up a lot in clinic and, for the most part, occurs due to dieting and childhood experiences. Dieting can lead to clean plate syndrome since it instils the belief that you are only permitted to eat at mealtimes. This injection of scarcity will encourage you to override your hunger, fullness, and satisfaction cues and finish the food on your plate because how could you leave food behind if you know you can't have any more until your next meal, no matter what? If scarcity is present, it's doubtful you will leave food on your plate, even if you're full. This is why honouring your fullness cues hinges critically on removing restrictions and allowing all foods in unconditionally.

Your childhood experiences can also impact the development of clean plate syndrome. Growing up in Ireland, two of the most common responses to a child not cleaning their plate were:

'Think about all those starving children in Africa.'

'It's a sin to waste food.'

This could be due to economic or other issues during childhood or it could result from ancestral experiences passed down from generation to generation. Intergenerational trauma, which is sometimes referred to as trans- or multigenerational trauma, is trauma that gets passed down from those who directly experienced it to subsequent generations. It often begins with a traumatic event affecting an individual or multiple family members, or a collective trauma affecting the whole community, or cultural, racial, ethnic, or other groups or populations (historical trauma). Irish people have historically experienced trauma around food scarcity, namely through the famines of the 1700s and 1800s and the rationing of food during the world wars of the 1900s – and unfortunately, many people today are suffering from food scarcity, so having an abundant supply of food is a privilege in itself.

This collective trauma of food scarcity is not exclusive to Ireland and affected millions of people in other European countries. The effects of this collective trauma can be passed down from generation to generation through the above statements from well-meaning parents. Like many other things we learn from parents or caregivers, this is rarely questioned until it's highlighted. This is nobody's fault and we must be cautious about placing blame on any one person. The topic of intergenerational trauma is a complex one, and this description is just to show that there may be other unconscious forces that affect your ability to stop eating when full – it is bigger than just you. The good news is that there's plenty you can do despite this. Here are some ways you can begin to tackle clean plate syndrome:

- Eliminate distractions when eating

- Eat slowly and mindfully

- Practise the pause (outlined later on in the chapter)

- Put your utensils down between bites

NOTE: This does not mean that you are committing to stopping eating, it simply gives you a chance to check in with your fullness cues.

- Remind yourself that 'the food will always be there' and you can eat whenever you want or need to

Value of food

This obstacle can show up as resistance to throwing out or not finishing all food due to historical beliefs around the value of money. It can originate in childhood, especially for those who grew up during difficult economic periods – for example, during the recessions of the 1980s and 2000s. Whether scarcity is self-inflicted through dieting, or as a result of financial scarcity, the impact is the same. Many of my clients who grew up during these eras remember not having money for the foods they really desired or food being scarce, which tends to leave a mark. After struggling with the value of food for some time, one of my clients developed some impressive wisdom concerning this. One day in a session, she said, 'My body is not a bin, and I'm done treating it like one.' The pride I felt for her at that moment, I can feel again right now as I share it with you. Nothing is more impressive to me than walking alongside my clients as they put time and energy into their healing and seeing them reap the benefits of doing so in moments like these.

Eating more than your body needs may be respecting economics but it is not necessarily respecting your body. Throwing food away may feel uncomfortable. If it does, remind yourself that you are looking after yourself and your health by doing so. Your body is one of the most valuable assets you own and will reward you when you treat it as such. For my clients who have struggled with this, it has helped them to pack any leftovers into a Tupperware box to have for later. Even if these leftovers are not eaten, it's often easier than throwing excess food straight into the bin.

Distraction
Eating while distracted is a surefire way of eating past comfortable fullness at the beginning of your journey of reconnecting with your hunger cues. Doing something else while eating can disrupt your ability to remain attuned to the body's signals. When you have fine-tuned the connection to your interoceptive awareness, you may be better able to eat while doing something else and still honour your fullness cues. However, when starting off, it's better to avoid distractions while eating where possible. These distractions could be eating while:

☐ Driving

☐ Working at your desk

☐ Reading

☐ Watching TV

☐ Listening to music

☐ Multitasking

It's not that doing these things are 'bad' (I love to eat in front of the TV sometimes too) and that you can never do them, but I'd advise against it where possible until you feel confident you can listen to your fullness cues despite the distraction.

Primal hunger
Eating from a stage of primal hunger is possibly one of the biggest obstacles to feeling your fullness. When you begin eating from a zero or one on the hunger scale, the need for nourishment supersedes the need to check in with fullness cues. Remember, it takes the body around twenty minutes to register that you are full. When you eat very fast, you miss the subtle cues of fullness entirely and end up feeling the effects of uncomfortable fullness a little while later. Willpower will never win against hunger; hunger will always win. Maintaining a regular eating pattern where possible and eating when subtly hungry will make it possible to honour your fullness cues when they arise.

Air food
Air food fills up the stomach but offers little sustenance. When you fill the tummy up with 'air food' — for example, popcorn, rice cakes, celery sticks — when you really need more food, it provides the illusion of fullness, which can be referred to as

'fake fullness'. This is probably something you can recognize from diet culture in the form of recommendations like having a glass of water or a coffee instead of food.

Fake fullness doesn't last very long, since you cannot trick the body into believing that you've given it what it needs. Eventually, the body will realize and send out hunger cues at an even greater intensity. When your body needs a meal, a snack won't do. This is why it's important to know the difference between meal hunger and snack hunger, so you can give your body the sustenance it requires. In general, meal hunger shows up when you experience hunger at an intensity of a 0–3 on the hunger scale; snack hunger is experienced at a 4 or 5.

Reconnecting with Your Fullness Cues

The hunger fullness scale discussed in Chapter 6 can help you reconnect with the subtle and more obvious signs of fullness. Ideally, you should finish eating around a six or seven on the scale. As I mentioned when we spoke about hunger, you may overeat sometimes and this is completely normal. We all overeat at times – there is no such thing as perfect eating. However, eating to the overfull stage regularly will not feel good in your body and will most likely make you feel sluggish and lethargic.

Consider the Staying Power

The nutritional components of a meal will have a substantial impact on how long you feel satiated afterwards. A filling meal will generally contain all three macronutrients: carbohydrate, protein, and fat. I will go into greater detail of what foods are contained within these categories in Part 3 of the book. Ideally, it will also contain fibre, which slows down the emptying of food from the stomach into the intestines, helping you feel fuller for longer. Fibre is found in complex carbohydrates, such as brown bread, pasta and rice, fruits and vegetables, and nuts and seeds. All of these add up to what can be called the 'staying power' of a meal. Some foods will fill you for longer than others. This doesn't mean that some foods are 'good' and others are 'bad'; it's simply information you can use to inform your future food choices.

Try some meals with all four elements (carbohydrate, fat, protein and fibre) and pay attention to how long you feel full. Then remove one or two of these components and do the same. How long do you feel full when only two or three of these components are present? This can be a fascinating exercise to help you consider the staying power of different meals.

Practise the Pause

To become aware of fullness cues, you will need to slow down and check in with them while eating. The exercise below will guide you through this, but it will be impossible to do if you are eating from a stage of primal hunger — trying this practice when gently hungry is imperative to its effectiveness.

Practising a pause while eating is *not* a commitment to stopping eating. Some clients have told me that stopping in the middle of their meal to check in felt like communicating that there was a need to stop or intentionally leave food on their plate, even if they had not yet hit comfortable fullness. This is not the intention of this exercise. The goal is simply to give yourself some time and space to check in with your fullness cues.

1. Check in with hunger level before eating
Use the hunger fullness scale to rate your hunger level before eating. Are you over-hungry — for example, a zero or one on the hunger fullness scale? If so, it might be a good idea to practise this at another time when you are starting to eat from a two to four on the scale.

2. Pause in the middle of eating
Take a pause while eating, for just ten to thirty seconds, and check in with taste and satiety by asking yourself the following questions. Taste check:

☐ How does the food taste?

☐ Is it still worthy of my taste buds?

☐ Am I still eating just because it's there?

Satiety check:

☐ What is my hunger or fullness level now?

☐ Am I still hungry?

☐ Am I unsatisfied?

☐ Is my hunger going away?

☐ Am I beginning to feel fullness?

After asking yourself these questions, you may decide to continue eating because you do not feel comfortably full or satisfied. Alternatively, you may discover that you are indeed comfortably full and satisfied and decide to stop eating. Remember, even if you decide to stop eating now, you can always continue eating again whenever you wish.

3. Check in with fullness level at the end
When you're finished eating, check in with your fullness level again and ask yourself these questions:

- ☐ Is the feeling of fullness pleasant, unpleasant, or neutral?

- ☐ Are you comfortably full?

- ☐ Did you surpass comfortable fullness?

- ☐ If you reached uncomfortable fullness, would you choose to feel this way again?

- ☐ If not, what would you do differently next time?

Approach any insights that arise with compassionate curiosity. Don't judge yourself if you overeat or overdo it; this is all information you can use for future experiences. Hitting the fullness level that feels 'just right' is a little like trying to hit a bullseye: it takes time and practice.

Affirmations

I am learning to identify what comfortable fullness feels like in my body.

I give myself permission to eat until comfortable fullness.

I am compassionate with myself when I overeat.

I am practising mindfulness with my meals.

I release the need to clean my plate.

The food will always be there; it's safe for me to stop eating when full.

Chapter 9:

Reconnecting with Your Emotions

When I speak about nourishment and meeting your needs, I don't just mean the physical or physiological needs that food satisfies; I'm also referring to meeting your emotional needs. How could you possibly be truly well and healthy if your emotional needs are being denied? If your emotional needs are not being met, food can fill the void, which is when people begin to experience issues with emotional eating. Reconnecting with your emotions and understanding the messages or unmet needs they are trying to communicate to you is vital in moving towards long-term health and well-being. Learning how to do this is an essential skill that will help to support your mental health. Regardless of whether or not you feel like you struggle with emotional eating, you will benefit from reconnecting with your emotions and understanding on a deeper level what messages they are trying to communicate to you. This chapter is for everyone, no matter how much or how little you struggle with your relationship with food.

What Is Emotional Eating?

Emotional eating gets a lot of bad press. It can be defined as using food to cope with, mask, or regulate abrupt changes in mood states. Every single person I have worked with in my clinic has experienced emotional eating at some point or another in the story of their relationship with food. Emotional eating is often demonized by diet culture and treated as a dragon that must be slayed. You do not have to completely rid yourself of emotional eating to have a healthy relationship with food. Instead, we should look at resolving emotional *over-eating*, since this often results in more problems than it solves.

Having an emotional connection to food makes sense. Newborn babies need to be held close when fed and they are comforted through the feeding process. This biological need for food is connected to a positive emotional experience. Then as we move through childhood, food is often given as a reward, a bribe, or in response to an emotion. Every time you have received food in response to a feeling of sadness, happiness, frustration, or anger – and it soothed you in the moment, the emotional connection with food was strengthened. This is not inherently bad, but we cannot rely solely on food to soothe us in times of distress. Food will not fix your feelings, and over-using it for this purpose can quickly turn food into a destructive rather than constructive coping strategy.

Emotional eating occurs on a continuum of intensity that begins at one end with mild sensory eating and finishes at the opposite end with numbing, anaesthetizing eating. If your version of emotional eating is for pleasure, comfort, or some-times a distraction, this doesn't necessarily indicate you have a problem with emotional eating. If food is the only thing that comes to mind to take care of yourself when you're experiencing uncomfortable emotions, you are regularly using food to distract yourself from these feelings, or you are sedating or punishing yourself with food, then you could likely benefit from working on this.

Physical and Emotional Hunger

It's important to be able to distinguish between physical and emotional hunger so you can define whether a physical or emotional need is calling out to be met when you experience an urge to eat. Physical hunger cannot be satisfied by anything other than food. Emotional hunger cannot be satisfied by food. Both types of hunger manifest differently.

Physical hunger:
- ☐ Comes on gradually and can be postponed

- ☐ Is satisfied by eating something

- ☐ Can be sated – you can stop eating when full

- ☐ Can be satisfied without guilt

Emotional hunger:
- ☐ Comes on suddenly and feels urgent

- ☐ Causes very specific cravings

- ☐ Cannot be easily sated – it's common to eat past fullness and feel uncomfortably full

☐ Cannot be completely satisfied by food, and you
feel guilt

Once you have identified whether it's physical or emotional
hunger you are experiencing, the next step is to meet those
physical or emotional needs.

Causes of Emotional Eating

There are certain things we can look out for that contribute
to emotional eating. Working through them one by one will
help you understand why you might be turning to food. There
are three leading causes.

1. Deprivation
Deprivation can manifest in a few ways — not eating enough
food regularly and consistently or through physical or mental
restriction. If your physiological needs for food are not being
met, the body will send out signals and hormones to ensure
those needs get met, as discussed in Chapter 6 when we spoke
about hunger. Food is the only solution to physical hunger. This
deprivation or scarcity mindset may end up feeling like
emotional eating, even though it's a normal and expected
reaction to not getting enough food or denying yourself what
you truly desire. Sometimes what we label as emotional eating
might be just hunger or a backlash from restriction.

2. Lack of self-care practices
Food can fill the void when you lack sufficient self-care practices, which include meeting your physical, mental, emotional,

spiritual, and future self-care needs. Say you have a friend or loved one who often comments on and judges the food you eat. If you do not set sufficient boundaries with this person, you may rebel by eating more of that food out of spite or eating it in secret. Rather than communicating what you need – for the comments to stop – you direct that frustration inwards towards yourself.

Another real-life example that comes up a lot, especially with people who have young families, is night-time eating. I know many of you will relate to that feeling of joy when you sit down in front of the TV with your favourite food after putting the kids to bed, or even just after a long, hard day at work. There's nothing wrong with doing this, but if you rely upon it for any particular reason, it can be a sign of emotional eating. I have worked with many clients who cannot seem to stop this behaviour – and for a good reason. It's often the only time they get for themselves in their day, and they don't want to give that up. This emotional eating will persist if they do not meet their own needs. If no time is carved out of the day for you, you will find it very difficult to give up the comfort food provides. Making time for yourself might mean asking for support or setting boundaries around work or home life, hence self-care. We will cover self-care in greater detail in Chapter 11.

3. Struggling to cope with emotions

The final cause of emotional eating lies in emotional regulation. Food may be your saviour if you struggle to cope with certain emotions. For example, if you struggle to cope with anger, biting on hard and crunchy foods may give you a release. If you struggle with sadness or loneliness, food may become a reliable friend to soothe you in those moments. First, please, please do not beat yourself up over this. Many people have not been given adequate tools to manage their emotions. But, luckily, this is something you can learn how to do. You can heal emotional overeating by developing more effective coping strategies and becoming friends with your feelings so you do not have to resort to food as often in an attempt to cope.

Discover Your Triggers

Everyone who struggles with emotional eating will have several situations or feelings that trigger the drive to overeat or use food to cope. Uncovering these will help you better understand yourself and develop more constructive ways to deal with the situation. If you are unsure how to begin uncovering your triggers for overeating, I suggest keeping an emotional eating journal. If you feel that keeping a food diary would be a triggering experience for you, it's worth remembering that you don't need to record precisely what is eaten during these times. You could simply write down the situation and the feelings that accompanied it. Here are a few examples of emotional triggers that could be a good starting point to your emotional eating journal:

Sadness — carbohydrates stimulate the production of serotonin, our 'feel good' hormone

Relaxation — using food as a means to rest or relieve stress

Procrastination — using food to delay a task

197

Anxiety – using food to calm yourself down

Lack of fulfilment – using food as a purpose

Reward – using food to reward yourself for a hard day

Distraction – using food to distract from uncomfortable emotions

Anger or frustration – using food as a release

Loneliness – using food as a friend

Joy – using food to celebrate

Boredom – eating as something to do

Is there anything on this list that resonates with you or that you recognize in yourself? As always, please approach this with curiosity instead of judgement. If you're interested in learning more about the triggers of emotional eating, I recommend *The Intuitive Eating Workbook*. It contains an entire chapter of exercises to help with emotional eating and is written by the founders of intuitive eating.[1] The goal here is not to judge yourself for using food in response to any of the above but to learn more about yourself in order to develop some constructive coping skills.

Deconstructing Emotional Eating

When a client comes to me after experiencing a bout of emotional eating or even binge eating, it's crucial to spend some time deconstructing the experience so that we can learn from it and bring those insights into future experiences.

It's not a good idea to completely avoid and push away the experience, to try and forget about it. I completely understand why people do this, especially if the incident was particularly distressing. However, when this happens, we fail to take any learnings from the experience and will most likely end up in the same situation the next time that it happens. In other words, avoiding it prevents us from using the experience to grow, and examining why we are emotionally overeating or binge eating is critical to healing. There are a few questions that I often ask my clients to help them do this. These are simple and easy to remember — think of the acronym HALT — so hopefully you can use them in your own struggles with this. Firstly, stop, take a breath, and then ask yourself:

H: Am I hungry?

A: Am I angry?

L: Am I lonely?

T: Am I tired?

I often share with my clients that the 'A' and the 'L' don't just stand for anger and loneliness. Instead, think of the 'A' as standing for emotions with an activated vibe, and the 'L' for those with a low vibe. For example, anger, anxiety, frustration, restlessness, and fear all have quite a visceral or 'activated' response in the body. Sadness, loneliness, vulnerability, grief, or disappointment are heavier emotions with a much lower vibration or corresponding feeling in the body.

If you identify that the overeating is indeed due to an emotional state, you may go a little further by asking yourself:

☐ How do I feel?

☐ What do I need?

By asking yourself these questions, either in the moment or in hindsight, you are becoming more connected to the true needs you may be trying to fill with food. It is only through this compassionate and curious questioning that you will reduce the frequency of emotional eating.

Reconnecting with Your Emotions

Reconnecting with and understanding the purpose of your emotions is an essential part of learning how to regulate and heal from emotional overeating. Your emotions are messengers; they educate, motivate, or illuminate. Emotions are fundamental — they communicate your needs to you. Every single emotion you experience has a purpose. Labelling emotions as positive or negative can fuel our desire to run away from the negative ones. But even these 'negative' emotions have an important message to tell us. When I first reframed my emotions as messengers, it completely transformed my relationship with them. Instead of seeing some of them as an experience I wanted to avoid, I began asking myself, 'What is this emotion trying to tell me?' This powerful reframing can give you bucketloads of information about what's going on within and therefore enable you to more effectively meet your emotional needs. Being emotionally healthy is not about being happy all the time. It's about being able to experience a range of emotions and be at ease with them, accepting them and letting them go.

Dancing with them as they ebb and flow. Here are some examples of what a range of emotions may be trying to communicate to you:

- ☐ Anger: helps us to stand up for ourselves, put boundaries in place, or protect ourselves or others in the face of threat

- ☐ Anxiety: alerts us to potential danger and is there to keep us safe

- ☐ Loneliness: a sign that we need to connect with others

- ☐ Sadness: a sign that we have lost something or someone that meant something to us, signalling that we need to take time to recuperate

- ☐ Guilt: a reminder that we are not living in alignment with our values and a sign to check in with our moral code

As you can see, each emotion above, no matter how uncomfortable, is trying to portray an important message and signal for further action. If we avoid certain emotions, we also miss out on the information they are trying to deliver to us.

Labelling Your Emotions

The first step in becoming reconnected to the messages your emotions are trying to deliver to you is to label them. How could you possibly reconnect with them if you're struggling to understand what it is you're feeling in the first place? Labelling your emotions requires a connection to the self and a fine-tuning of your interoceptive awareness, which can be cultivated through practising mindfulness, as we discussed in Chapter 5. When I teach my clients how to label their emotions, I share the benefits of using both a 'top-down' and a 'bottom-up' approach. The 'top-down' approach requires the cognitive labelling of emotions primarily utilizing the mind. The 'bottom-up' approach uses the physical sensations in the body to guide you to the appropriate label. Every emotion has a corresponding physical sensation in the body.

Emotions are simply energy in motion. Think of a time when you felt nervous, anxious, or excited. Think about how you might feel going into a job interview, going on a first date, or presenting to a large crowd of people. In these nervous moments, you may feel butterflies in the tummy or a sense of nausea or upset. This is because of the direct connection between the brain and the gut via the vagus nerve – what is experienced in the mind is felt in the gut and vice versa. When we pay attention to the physical sensations that accompany our emotions, they can provide us with vital information that we may not be otherwise aware of. It may be that when you become connected to the physical sensations in the body, you notice emotions there before you even realize that you're feeling them.

I was having a conversation with a friend one day when, all of a sudden, I experienced an immediate sensation of coldness in my body in response to something she said. My limbs became heavy, my heart was in my mouth, and it felt like all the blood had left my body. This was fear. I recognized it immediately because I had already done some personal work on connecting with the physical sensations of my own emotions. On further exploration, I couldn't tie this feeling of fear to any one thing in particular, but if the body was signalling it, it was there nonetheless. The body doesn't lie, but the mind often will. Since the body doesn't have a mechanism for lying to you or covering something up with reasoning or justifications, you can trust that what you are feeling in your body is true. By honouring the physical sensations I was feeling in my body at that moment and understanding how closely related they were to fear, I could not deny that it was indeed fear that I was experiencing. This was the start of some personal exploration, which led to significant changes in my life. And this, dear reader, is the power of connecting with your emotions. Developing and honing this skill has the ability to change the trajectory of your life. Emotions provide you with valuable information — they should never be ignored.

Here are some of the physical sensations that may accompany specific categories of emotions. Remember that these may feel different in your body, and your experience of feeling these emotions may bring up other sensations for you — we are all unique.

- ☐ Anger: tight jaw, racing heart, feeling hot, clenching

- ☐ Fear: frozen, trembling, fidgety, unsteady

- ☐ Happiness: energetic, awake, still, warm

- ☐ Surprise: speechless, jaw drop, sweaty palms, jumpy

☐ Sadness: empty, heaviness, slow heartbeat, curling up

☐ Disgust: nausea, face-scrunching, shuddering, lump in the throat

Feeling Your Feelings

I know it sucks to feel some of the emotions we encounter throughout our lives. Who would want to feel sadness, frustration, or grief? But experiencing these emotions is part of living a human life — suffering is unavoidable. None of us can predict the suffering that may come our way, but we can learn to approach these emotions with compassion and soften around them when they arrive. To do that, we need to learn to feel our feelings rather than run away from them. We need to sit into them and allow them to pass through us. The more you run away from certain emotions, the more terrifying they become, and the more resistant you will become to feeling them.

I know this is easier said than done, but it's essential. When we don't allow ourselves to feel our feelings, they don't go away. They bury themselves deep within the body and eventually manifest in physical symptoms, sometimes chronic diseases. As the saying goes, disease is dis-ease. At the heart of every destructive coping mechanism there is the illusion that we can control our emotions; we can't. They are a part of life and an important part at that! Having said that, emotions are temporary. They come and go. It's not unusual for a human being to feel a rainbow of different emotions in a 24-hour period. Just because you feel an emotion right now does not mean you will feel that way forever. The only guarantee in life is impermanence. The same can be said for our emotions.

If you struggle with feeling your feelings, it can be helpful to compare your emotions to waves. Imagine you're standing on the beach looking out at the water. You see a wave gathering speed far off in the distance. As it comes closer to you, it gathers momentum, getting higher and higher, until it hits a peak and then crashes and subsides. This is exactly how we experience emotions. Learning to surf the wave rather than getting dragged underneath is a skill known as emotional regulation. If you have not been taught how to emotionally regulate, it makes sense to be scared of feeling your feelings. The good news is that you can hone your emotional regulation muscle through practice. You can do this by working on expanding your coping skills toolkit, which we will discuss in the following section. If you feel like you struggle with emotional eating, learning to feel your feelings and emotionally regulate will play a key role in resolving this issue.

Expanding Your Coping Skills Toolkit

There's a sneaky way that diet culture operates when it comes to emotional eating, and that's to brand it as a bad thing that must be abolished. In reality, emotional eating is a normal and expected part of a healthy relationship with food. We all emotionally eat from time to time, and attempting to stop it entirely is a battle you will never win. And why should you even try? Eating for joy, sadness, frustration, and so on can be a pleasurable and soothing experience. Emotional eating only becomes problematic when food is the dominant or only coping strategy in your toolkit and is therefore overused to the point of overeating or bingeing. Most people who struggle with emotional eating are doing the best that they can with the resources they have to hand.

At the end of the day, food is giving you something that leads you to turn to it again and again. Rather than criticizing yourself for doing this, maybe even when you know it's causing you problems, can you remain open and curious about what needs it might be meeting for you? Once you get an insight into the needs food might be fulfilling, you will be better able to meet those needs with a coping strategy that is even more beneficial to you than food. Compassion is essential here — be kind to yourself as you explore this. In the interim, the goal is not to rip away a coping strategy that may be essential for you to survive or make it through different emotional states. To heal from an emotional dependency on food, you will need to expand your toolkit of coping skills, then slowly wean yourself off food by adding these new strategies into your life when uncomfortable emotions hit. Anita Johnson, the author of *Eating in the Light of the Moon*, tells a beautiful story demonstrating this process in her book. Imagine you were to fall into a river; you cannot swim and you have no life jacket. You are trying very hard to keep afloat, but the strength of the river and your lack of swimming skills are causing you to drown. All of a sudden, a huge log floats toward you. You grab onto it and hold on for dear life until you come to a place where the water is calm. You can see the shore in the near distance, but your lack of swimming skills is holding you back. You cannot swim there while still holding onto the log, but you have no confidence that you can make it on your own. You need to build up the swimming skills you need before you can confidently let go of that log that once saved your life. So, you begin to practise floating by very slowly and carefully, letting go of the log. As described by Anita:

> When you start to sink, you grab back on. Then you let go of the log and practice treading water, and when you get tired, hold on once again. After a while, you practice swimming around the log once, twice, ten times, twenty times, a hundred times, until you gain the strength and confidence you need to swim to shore. Only then do you completely let go of the log.[2]

As she explains, simply letting go of the log may not be the best course of action, especially if there is a dependency on it to survive. What if you were to let go of the log and then realize halfway across the river that you didn't have the strength to either make it back to the log or onward to the shore? You'd be kind of screwed, right? People can feel foolish when they realize they are still clinging to disordered eating behaviours when they know how much distress they are causing. Still, perhaps these behaviours have helped you to deal with difficult times in your life when you didn't have any other alternative. Rather than condemning the behaviour, I invite you to honour its role in your life. Doing so allows you to create the space and compassion required to explore the purpose it has provided you. Lean into it rather than recoiling from it. When you do this, deep learning can occur.

To replace the log with a more constructive coping strategy, you must first develop the skills required to replace the function it provided. Once you develop these skills, you will find that they are more effective than the disordered eating behaviour and choose these instead. You can then let go of the log, confident in your ability to make it to shore, thanks to these new-found skills that will keep you afloat. Your confidence will grow, but it requires time and practice.

When I speak about expanding a coping-skills toolkit with my clients, I often refer to building a 'Mary Poppins's bag' of coping skills. Having one or two tools is not enough; we need many options to draw on at different times, depending on our needs. I had a client whose primary purpose in working with me was to heal her emotional dependency on food. There were, of course, lots of other elements that were feeding into this dependency that needed to be worked through in our one-to-one sessions, but a turning point in the process happened when we began to build out her 'Mary Poppins's bag' of coping skills. Rather than removing food as a coping strategy during difficult times, we added other skills instead. So, for example, instead of simply numbing out with food in front of the TV, we added journalling as an adjunctive practice. Journalling helped her to gain insight and clarity into what was going on in her inner landscape, but accepting that food was still needed alongside it, at least for that time, allowed her to explore this new coping strategy with less struggle and resistance. We created some safety alongside discomfort. Over time, her dependency on food lessened to the point where she no longer needed it to cope emotionally.

To get started on expanding your own toolkit of coping skills, pull out a piece of paper and write down all the things that help you deal with challenging times or situations. If you are completely lost, don't worry. Below is a list of alternative coping strategies, some of which may work better for you than others. Building your own toolkit of coping skills may take a little bit of trial and error as you uncover what does and does not work for you. Having a coping-skills toolkit is closely related to self-care, which will be covered in Chapter 11. Creating a system of self-care in your life will also support you in coping with uncomfortable moments or situations:

- ☐ Talking to someone you trust
- ☐ Therapy
- ☐ Breathing techniques
- ☐ Muscle relaxation techniques
- ☐ Yoga
- ☐ Meditation
- ☐ Movement/exercise
- ☐ Using positive affirmations
- ☐ Doing things that bring you joy
- ☐ Accepting uncertainty
- ☐ Helpful distraction
- ☐ Expressing your feelings

- ☐ Talking a walk in nature
- ☐ Journalling
- ☐ Asking for hugs
- ☐ Reading
- ☐ Listening to music
- ☐ Sitting with your feelings
- ☐ Gratitude
- ☐ Self-compassion
- ☐ Setting boundaries and saying no
- ☐ Spending time with friends
- ☐ Making time for fun
- ☐ Travelling
- ☐ Making art
- ☐ Connecting with your community
- ☐ Having fulfilling work
- ☐ Rest
- ☐ Getting enough sleep
- ☐ Mindful awareness
- ☐ Crying
- ☐ Learning something new

- ☐ Playing with pets
- ☐ Dancing
- ☐ Buying yourself flowers
- ☐ Clean bedlinen
- ☐ Wearing comfortable clothes
- ☐ Cuddling up to a blanket or teddy
- ☐ Taking holidays

Affirmations

I hold space for all my emotions and respond with compassionate curiosity.

I accept my emotions and allow them to pass through me.

My feelings are real and valid.

I listen to the messages my emotions are giving me.

All emotions are temporary.

This too shall pass.

PART 3: RE-ESTABLISH

Re-establish health-promoting behaviours from this new perspective that you've developed by first removing anything that does not serve you and then reconnecting with the needs of your mind and body.

Before We Begin

So now that we have removed the diet mentality and reconnected with the mind, body, and self, how do we begin to
embrace health in a way that isn't damaging? The thing is,
dieting is not healthy: it's harmful behaviour — even when it's
masquerading as a healthy 'lifestyle change'. By now, you know
that dieting has many negative consequences. On the surface,
it may sometimes look like it's contributing to health, but when
we dig deeper, it's a wolf dressed up in sheep's clothing and
leaves us worse off than when we started. So, we need to
embrace a new way of looking at health, that doesn't have
even a *sniff* of diet culture about it.

There are many ways that you can begin improving your
health without ever focusing on weight loss. That might seem
radical, but really, if you are doing all the right things for
your health and your weight does not change, what more
can you do? The focus of this final part of the book will be
on showing you what you can do for your health without the

caveat of weight loss being a progress marker. At the end of the day, we could all eat the same and exercise the same but we would still not look the same as one another.

When I work with my clients, either one-on-one or through my online programmes, when they reach the stage of readiness for re-establishing their health-promoting behaviours, I am not interested in whether those behaviours do or do not lead to weight loss. That's because, frankly, weight is not an indicator of health. You could live in a large body and be healthier than someone living in a small body. Rather than focusing on something you cannot wholly control – i.e. weight – it can be empowering to direct your energy towards things you can. There are many ways you can start to do this, which I have integrated into what I call the wheel of health. This integrates the five pillars of health that I often speak about with clients. Each pillar is equally important, which is why we look at it in a rounded manner:

WHEEL OF HEALTH

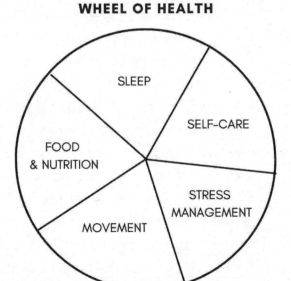

Health is about so much more than the food on your plate. I take an integrated approach when helping people to improve their health by looking at their lives as a whole. It's not always obvious when certain behaviours or circumstances are disrupting your ability to look after yourself. This is where nutrition counselling can be extremely helpful to help you figure that out.

So, what do healthy behaviours look like? Here is a little snapshot:

☐ Eating lots of fruits and vegetables

☐ Moving your body regularly

☐ Setting boundaries at home, work, or school

☐ Spending time with people you love

☐ Taking time to rest

☐ Spending time alone

☐ Reflecting on your life

☐ Practising gratitude

☐ Going to therapy

☐ Asking for help

I could go on, but the point is that health is unique to each of us and expansive in nature. It can look very different from person to person based on their life circumstances. As always, I believe that you have a unique perspective and are the expert of your own body. You know what makes you feel good, and if you have yet to discover what does, you can now embark on an exciting journey to figure that out.

Diet Culture Masquerading as a Health Goal

When my clients feel ready to embrace health-promoting behaviours, they often come up against the question of whether they are genuinely doing this for health reasons or if some sneaky weight-loss messages are driving their desire. It's important to check in with your intention by asking yourself why you are making these changes in your life. What outcome is most important to you? Then ask yourself:

Would I do this even if it never changed my body size or shape?

This will quickly help you understand if your decision to embrace health-promoting behaviours is grounded in diet culture or a pure intention for health. If you answer no to this question, it might indicate that you have a little more work to do in the remove and reconnect stages before moving on to the final re-establish phase.

Cultivating New Habits

Before we get into the five pillars of health in detail, let's talk a little about cultivating new habits, which is what you will be doing when implementing the strategies discussed in the following chapters. Habits are hard to create or break, but doing so is 100 per cent possible — with a plan. Throwing yourself into a new routine without a plan is a recipe for disaster. Planning is crucial for success. Many of my clients fear planning because of how closely related it feels to dieting. The difference here is your intention. Planning with a compassionate mindset allows you to be flexible with your plan, whereas when planning is hooked to diet culture, it is often rigid: there is no space for flexibility.

In my Setting Sustainable Wellness Goals workshop, I teach people how to set wellness goals that last, and one of the key strategies I teach is the four Ws. The four Ws can help you to form new habits and get clear on how to make that happen:

- ☐ **What** is the habit you would like to achieve or eliminate?

- ☐ **Why** do you want it? Look at instant and future reasons why.

- ☐ **When** are you going to do this? Get specific with time and for how long. Make sure it's achievable, and prepare to be flexible with this.

- ☐ **Where** will it happen?

Be on the lookout for any barriers that arise and approach them with curiosity instead of judgement. Ask yourself, 'What can I learn from this?' Do not give up if you don't manage to engage in the habit despite your planning — this is normal. You are trying; be compassionate with yourself. It may just signify that you need to tweak your plan and try again. Ask yourself, 'How could I do better next time?' Start small and build on your habits — small actions sustained over time always have more impact than significant actions that aren't. I suggest focusing on one change at a time for a period of two to three weeks. When that habit feels embedded, move onto the next. Slow and steady wins the race here. Anything worth having takes time. Let's begin.

Chapter 10:

Sleep

How happy are you with your current sleep pattern? Would you say you get enough or that your sleep is of high quality? If your answer is no, you're not alone. Sleep is possibly one of the most important but underrated aspects of health and well-being. Without sleep, everything becomes more challenging, even the simplest responsibilities, not to mention the behaviours that require more commitment, such as eating well or regular movement. Engaging in health-promoting behaviours requires energy, and sleep plays an essential role in topping up your energy stores. We are all aware of how difficult life becomes when your sleep is poor and your body is running on empty as a result. It can affect your mood, energy, and relationships. It's harder to concentrate, to face and resolve daily challenges, and to generally get on with the demands of day-to-day life – let alone work on improving your health! Survival becomes the goal. How can you thrive if you're struggling to survive on poor-quality sleep? A past client of mine was able to link all of her issues with food back to poor-quality sleep, and once this was resolved, these issues fell away. Needless to say, time to sleep and rest is a non-negotiable for her now!

I understand that this may be a sensitive subject for some of you, especially if you struggle with insomnia, have a young family, or are dealing with other uncontrollable factors affecting your sleep quantity or quality. I am not delusional enough to believe that simply reading this chapter will solve any of these issues, but as I always say, when it comes to your health, let's focus on what we can control rather than what we can't. There is liberation in letting go and surrendering to those things you (honestly) cannot control while taking responsibility for what you can. There are many amazing books that cover the intricacies of sleep, such as *Why We Sleep* by the renowned neuroscientist Matthew Walker, if you'd like to do a deep dive into the science — this book is not one of those.[4] The aim of this chapter is to provide you with actionable, ready-to-implement tools and strategies to help you begin to improve your sleep quality.

The Importance of Sleep

Good sleep is essential for physical, mental, and emotional health. Sleep is not just a time for rest; it's also critical for the body to repair and regenerate. It is an incredibly complex process that affects virtually all systems in the body. The fact that almost all animal species need to sleep gives us clues as to how important it is. When you get enough sleep, your brain is better able to concentrate and make decisions. Your hunger and fullness cues are better regulated, and you feel more energized and alert. In adults, a lack of sleep has been associated with a wide range of adverse health consequences, including cardiovascular problems[1], a weakened immune system[2], and a higher risk of type 2 diabetes.[3]

So how much sleep do you need? This depends on the individual, as the ideal number of hours of sleep a person needs a night can vary. However, the National Sleep Foundation guidelines advise that healthy adults need between seven and nine hours of sleep per night. Babies, young children, and teens need even more sleep to enable their growth and development. People over 65 should get seven to eight hours per night. These are optimum ranges. However, there's some wiggle room on either side for an 'acceptable', though still not optimal, amount of sleep. This acceptable range of sleep for adults ranges from six to ten hours. Any more or less than this, and you can suffer the effects of inadequate sleep or oversleeping.

What's Affecting Your Sleep?

The issue of inadequate or low-quality sleep comes up often with my clients, yet many of them will tell me how important a good night's sleep is to their daily routine. It's clear to them that it needs to be addressed, but they struggle to figure out how exactly to do that and what advice to follow. Sleep is a huge topic and it can feel overwhelming when you pay Dr Google a visit and see the sheer quantity of information and resources available. If there's one thing we all know about sleep, it's that overthinking it only makes matters worse! To avoid this overwhelm when it comes up as an issue with my clients, I take a very personalized approach to help them overcome it.

This is because inadequate sleep is a personal issue, and therefore the solution needs to also be personal. Just like any other strategies and topics I've discussed here, becoming your own expert is central to the process. That is not to say that knowledge and education around sleep is not important — it absolutely is — but only when layered on top of a connection to your personal situation and what might be causing it.

Each person who encounters sleep problems may have a different set of barriers that are affecting their sleep and a different set of behaviours that are maintaining the issue. When I take a personalized approach with my clients, before providing any advice on the issue, we try to figure out, as a team, what these barriers and maintenance behaviours are. Problems with sleep quality or quantity are not usually an isolated issue, especially for people who at one time slept soundly.

For example, a past client of mine, who was going through a stressful time in his life, was finding it harder to fall asleep at night than ever before. Stress and anxiety are common triggers for sleep problems. His two young children would also wake at different times during the night, which added further insult to injury. The issue he was having with falling asleep was leading to more stress and anxiety. To try and help the situation, he began having a small glass of wine before bed. This gave him some much-needed reprieve from the stress he was experiencing, which helped him to fall asleep. But as with all substances, over time, he needed more to get the same effect. Soon, the alcohol was causing sleep disturbances and he would wake up groggy in the morning only to have another stressful day and then rely upon the wine for sleep in the evening. It was a vicious cycle.

This is a perfect illustration of how an issue with sleep is often not an isolated issue. There can be many external and individual factors that affect it. In this case, the barriers that were causing my client's sleep issues were his young children and the stress and anxiety caused by external factors. Once a client's barriers are uncovered, I categorize them into controllable and uncontrollable factors to decide what to focus on going forward. In this case, the sleep schedules of young children are often uncontrollable and unpredictable. Stress and anxiety are issues that can be tackled. The maintenance behaviour for my client was alcohol consumption, which was enlisted to try to cope with the stress, anxiety, and lack of sleep. Whenever I uncover maintenance behaviours with a client, I approach them with non-judgemental curiosity and compassion. That goes for you too! Most people are doing the best that they can to cope, and judging yourself upon the uncovering of these behaviours will not help. In this particular case, working on stress management techniques and building a sleep ritual personal to him was key to his sleep recovery. I'm happy to report that this client is now sleeping and thriving as a result!

So I encourage you to first try and uncover your own barriers and maintenance behaviours before implementing any sleep strategies. This will help you to find the true cause of your issues with sleep. Try asking yourself:

☐ What do I feel is causing my issues with sleep?

☐ Am I enlisting any behaviours to cope that are maintaining the issue?

If this is difficult to do alone, I highly recommend reaching out to a suitable professional who can help you uncover these barriers and maintenance behaviours.

Ten Tips for Better Sleep

There are many things you can do to begin improving your sleep, which I have compiled into ten tips, after being inspired from reading *Why We Sleep*. Keep these ten tips in mind as you work to improve your sleep routine:

1. Stick to a sleep schedule. Try to go to bed and wake up at the same time each day, creating an effective sleep pattern. Sleeping later on days off or on weekends won't fully make up for a lack of sleep during the week and will make it harder to wake up earlier on Monday morning. You can use an alarm for bedtime, just like you do for the morning. This is my first tip because it's the most important.

2. Avoid late-afternoon napping. Naps can help make up for lost sleep, but if taken after 3 p.m., they can make falling asleep harder at night.

3. Be conscious of what you're consuming close to bedtime, primarily stimulants such as caffeine, nicotine and alcohol, along with large meals and beverages. Coffee, certain teas, colas and choc- olate contain caffeine, and it can take as long as eight hours for their effects to wear off fully.

Drinking coffee late in the afternoon can wreak havoc on getting to sleep at night. Nicotine can cause smokers to sleep very lightly and wake too early in the morning because of nicotine withdrawal. Alcohol may help you relax before bedtime, but heavy consumption robs you of REM sleep, the phase of sleep that plays an important role in dreaming, memory, emotional processing and healthy brain development. It can also cause wakefulness during the night when its effects wear off. Finally, try not to consume large meals and beverages too close to bedtime. If you are hungry, by all means, have a snack, but large meals can cause indigestion, which interferes with sleep. Too much fluid before bedtime will also cause wakefulness to urinate.

4. Try not to exercise too late in the day. Exercise taken less than two to three hours before your bedtime can interrupt sleep by energizing the mind and body.

5. Expose yourself to natural daylight for at least thirty minutes each day. The right sunlight exposure is key to regulating daily sleep patterns. If possible, wake up with the sun or use very bright lights in the morning. Sleep experts recommend that, if you have problems falling asleep, you should get an hour of exposure to morning sunlight and dim the lights before bedtime.

6. Talk to your healthcare provider to see whether any of your medications might be contributing to your sleep problems or insomnia. Some commonly prescribed heart, blood pressure, or asthma medications, as well as some over-the-counter and herbal remedies for coughs, colds, or allergies, can disrupt sleep patterns. Ask whether they can be taken at other times during the day or early in the evening.

7. Take a hot bath or shower before bed. The drop in body temperature afterwards may help you feel sleepy, and the bath can help you relax and slow down, preparing you for a good night's sleep.

8. Relax before bed. Make sure to prioritize time at the end of the day to unwind. A relaxing activity, such as reading or listening to music, should be part of your bedtime ritual.

9. Be conscious of gadgets, temperature and light in the bedroom. Dim the lights, maintain a cool bedroom, and remove any gadgets, such as a TV, mobile phone or computer. These gadgets can be a distraction and deprive you of well-needed sleep. Blue light emitted from these appliances suppresses the body's release of melatonin, a hormone that makes us feel sleepy. If you have an alarm clock in your room, turn the clock's face out of view so you don't worry about

NIAMH ORBINSKI

the time while trying to fall asleep. Having a comfortable mattress, pillow and bedlinen can also help promote a good night's sleep.

10. Don't lie in bed awake. If you find yourself still awake after staying in bed for more than twenty minutes, don't toss and turn, get up and move. Get up and do some relaxing activity until you feel sleepy. The anxiety of not being able to sleep can make it harder to fall asleep, so try to tackle this, rather than lying in bed awake.

Creating a Sleep Ritual

Creating a sleep ritual or routine that sets you up for a good night's sleep can be incredibly supportive if you struggle with sleep quantity or quality. Sleep rituals are very individual – what works for me may not work for you. This is often referred to as 'sleep hygiene': having a bedroom environment and daily routines that promote consistent, uninterrupted sleep. Having a hard time falling asleep, experiencing frequent sleep disturbances, and suffering daytime sleepiness are the most telling signs of poor sleep hygiene. An overall lack of consistency in sleep quantity or quality can also be a symptom of poor sleep hygiene. Before creating your sleep ritual, you may want to try out some of the tips mentioned in the previous section to explore if making any of those changes impacts your sleep. If so, I recommend adding these to your sleep ritual to create your own sleep hygiene checklist. In general, there are four categories that can contribute to an effective sleep ritual:

1. Follow a sleep schedule

Going to bed or waking up at the same time every day of the week helps your ability to fall asleep when you want to. Also, a regular schedule helps to sync your circadian rhythm, which dictates when you feel sleepy or awake. Of course, there will be times when your sleep schedule will vary, but this should be the exception, not the rule:

- ☐ Have a fixed sleep and wake-up time

- ☐ Prioritize sleep

- ☐ Make gradual adjustments if changing your sleep schedule

- ☐ Don't overdo it with naps — keep them short and limited to the early afternoon

2. Create a relaxing bedtime routine

A bedtime routine carried out each night can teach the mind that it's time for sleep and to associate certain behaviours with getting ready to rest. Reinforcing the signals that it's time to sleep can reduce the likelihood of having trouble sleeping once you hit the hay. Here are some things to try just before you head to bed:

- ☐ Unplugging from electronics (do this thirty to sixty minutes before bedtime)

- ☐ Gentle stretching or meditation

- ☐ Breathing exercises

☐ Reading

☐ Listening to soft music

☐ Gentle, calming scents

☐ Putting aside thirty minutes for relaxation

☐ Keeping a consistent routine – for example, putting on pyjamas, then brushing teeth, facial cleansing, and so on

3. Optimize your bedroom environment

Your sleep environment is key for effective sleep hygiene. To fall asleep quickly and easily, your bedroom will need to emanate calm, peace, and tranquillity. What makes a bedroom feel this way will vary from person to person but here are some things to try:

☐ Invest in a comfortable mattress and pillow

☐ Ensure you enjoy the touch and feel of your bedding

☐ Be mindful of the colours you choose for your bedding – are they soft and calming or loud and busy?

☐ Block out the light

☐ Keep the room temperature cool

☐ Dim the lights and avoid harsh, bright lighting

☐ Subdue nearby sources of sound

☐ Try calming scents such as lavender, either dropped onto your pillow or released through a diffuser

4. Cultivate daily healthy habits

Healthy sleep starts before you hit the bed. The way that you live your life during the day will affect the way you sleep, so making improvements to your daily habits will help you sleep better at night. Therefore, all the content discussed in this final section of the book will contribute to a good night's sleep. Here are some pointers to keep in mind:

☐ Move your body regularly

☐ Be conscious of caffeine intake, especially late in the afternoon

☐ Manage your stress levels

☐ Maintain a regular eating pattern

☐ Be conscious of eating meals too close to bedtime

☐ Spend time outdoors

☐ Reduce alcohol consumption

☐ Curb smoking

☐ Use your bed for two things only — sleep and sex

Affirmations

My mind and body are ready to rest.

I let go of all that I cannot control.

It is safe to put my thoughts on hold while I sleep.

I choose to give my body the gift of restful sleep.

I am working on my sleep habits.

I release all tension from my mind and body

Chapter 11:

Self-Care

When you hear the word 'self-care', what comes to mind? When I first heard this word, I associated it with indulgence — getting your nails done, treating yourself to a weekend away, or spending some time at a spa. Yes, self-care is all these things, but it's also much more. Self-care has been packaged as a commodity, but the most important aspects of it cannot be purchased. No amount of bubble baths and spa visits will make up for a lack of basic self-care practices. When you embark on a journey of improving your health and well-being, taking a long, hard look at your self-care practices is non-negotiable. You cannot improve your health for the better without considering self-care. It's a crucial part of feeling your best. Developing a consistent self-care practice to become your best self will require a connection to the self and a commitment to honouring the needs of your mind and body. This chapter on self-care comes before we speak about food and nutrition because without first establishing a self-care practice, fuelling your body well will feel like an impossible task.

If I asked you how you were currently doing with self-care on a scale of one to ten, what would your answer be? What do you currently do to take care of yourself? Are you happy with your responses, or do you feel you could improve? Self-care is a critical foundation for rebuilding your relationship with food and rediscovering your intuitive eater. Most of us could do with improving our self-care practices. The extent to which we engage with self-care will also change with time, based on life circumstances. To stay on top of self-care will require lifelong check-ins with yourself. Checking in with yourself and your needs in this way, alongside committing time and energy to self-care, will improve your life on so many different levels.

What Actually Is Self-Care?

Essentially, self-care is anything you deem a necessary action to take care of yourself after tuning into the needs of your mind and body. This will not always be 'hedonic self-care', the type that is pleasurable but fleeting. Since your mental, emotional, physical, and spiritual needs can vary daily, so will your self-care needs. Self-care could look like going to bed early when you feel tired. It could be pushing yourself to exercise because it makes you feel good, but it could also look like changing into your pyjamas after a long day at work to relax and watch Netflix. Self-care will look different depending on the individual and their needs; it's a highly personal practice. And it is also a daily practice. You wouldn't brush your teeth once or twice and expect healthy teeth for the rest of your life. To have healthy teeth and gums, you must brush your teeth twice daily, every day, for life. Once this becomes a habit, it's just part of your daily routine. It's the same with self-care. It doesn't have to become another to-do list you strive to complete; instead, a self-care practice becomes part of how you show up for yourself every day. It becomes a lens through which you experience and respond to life.

Suzy Reading has a great definition of self-care:

Self-care is health care. It is nourishing all layers of your being — your mental health, your physical health, and your emotional health, all of which are inextricably linked . . . self-care is something that nurtures you right now, and promotes your health in the future, nourishing your 'future self.'[1]

An important part of this definition is that self-care involves nurturing your current self *and* looking after your future self. This is a really useful tool to check whether you're actually practising meaningful self-care. It encourages us to consider the short- and the long-term consequences of our actions. Looking after your future self might mean prioritizing things that aren't entirely pleasant, such as setting boundaries, having difficult conversations, or letting go of something you don't want to let go of in order to make space for new energy and growth. It may mean sitting through therapy and addressing things that feel uncomfortable to confront but are necessary for long-term growth and healing. If you believe self-care must mean feeling good in the present moment, you will miss out on satisfying your actual needs in service to your future self; therefore, an opportunity for growth will pass you by. Committing to a consistent self-care practice can make you happier, healthier, and more aligned with your values and the person you want to show up as in your life. This may require you to challenge deep-seated belief systems and patterns that have developed throughout your life.

If you did not grow up with a caregiver who modelled the importance of self-care, developing this skill may involve constructing a new definition of what it means to care for oneself. I often see a pattern in clinic, particularly in my female clients, of believing it's honourable to put yourself last and prioritize the people you love. This is usually something they have learned since childhood from watching a parent or grandparent. Yes, you should, of course, prioritize the people you love, but not at the expense of yourself. You cannot pour from an empty cup. Only when your own self-care needs are met can you look after others without feeling depleted or resentful. This is the ideal scenario.

There may of course, be certain circumstances that make it hard to look after your own needs. For example, you may be a single parent, you could be looking after or caring for loved ones who are sick or disabled or you could be going through a period of your life where there are extra demands placed on you. If this is the case for you, I suggest clarifying what your self-care non-negotiables are. That is, the things that are absolutely crucial to looking after yourself. For a client of mine who had four young children, this for her was having time alone to shower. This is simple, but can have a big impact. The following sections will help further with this. You can only do your best. Be gentle with yourself.

Your self-care needs can be divided into four categories: physical, mental and emotional, spiritual, and future. All these categories are related — how we act in one category will impact how we feel in another. For example, setting boundaries around time spent at work (mental and emotional self-care) will enable you the space to allocate to movement or exercise (physical self-care). Reflecting on the meaning and purpose of your life (spiritual self-care) can help to clarify the relationships you would like to dedicate energy to that support this (mental and emotional self-care). Making time to batch cook some extra portions of your favourite meal (future self-care) will help to nourish you during busy periods when you don't have the time to cook (physical self-care). This last one is a particular favourite of mine that I often employ in my own life. I will regularly thank my past self for looking after my future self when I go to the freezer and find a home-cooked meal I made weeks ago. There is no greater joy, and I feel like I've won the day when it happens! The following table shows some more examples of what looking after your physical, mental and emotional, spiritual, and future self-care needs might look like:

Physical	Mental and Emotional	Spiritual	Future
Food	Therapy	Prayer	Alone time

Movement	Relationships	Mindfulness and meditation	Eating enough fruit and vegetables
Hydration	Boundaries	Yoga	Choosing foods that make you feel well
Health check-ups	Making time for fun	Seeing the beauty in everyday things	Prioritizing movement
Taking holidays	Making time for rest	Reflecting on life	Sitting with the discomfort of setting boundaries
Wearing comfortable clothes	Journalling	Spending time in nature	Being mindful of caffeine/ sugar/fat intake
Adequate sleep	Hobbies	Connection to a higher power	Prepping food in advance for busy periods

This is by no means an exhaustive list, but it should give you some ideas as to what I mean when discussing these four categories of self-care. Your self-care practice is yours to develop — unique to you and your life circumstances. The intensity of your self-care practice will also ebb and flow in response to life; sometimes, you may need more self-care than others. If you are going through stress, burnout, grief, loss, or a transition in life, self-care can be the balm that soothes you during these challenging times and makes them easier to move through. Only you will know the level of self-care you require at any given time. Your understanding of this comes from connecting to your inner expert and being consciously aware of your ever-changing needs, which we discussed in Chapter 5. To be truly connected to your self-care needs will require consistent monitoring of your inner landscape to assess what it is your mind and body are calling out for.

The Self-Care Fire

I first learnt about the self-care fire analogy from my friend Robyn Taaffe, who I like to call the self-care queen. We were running a workshop together on overcoming emotional over-eating and I fell in love with the analogy she used to describe self-care, and so have many of my clients since (thanks, Robyn).

When you light a fire, you need a multitude of fuel sources: little sticks to catch the flame, medium-size branches to help it gain momentum, and large logs when the fire is big and strong. If you place a large log on top of a fire that hasn't caught or only has embers in the hearth, it will not make the fire any stronger. In fact, it will probably put it out! We can apply this analogy to self-care by reminding ourselves that there are little sticks, branches, and logs of self-care and that all of these are equally important to have in your toolkit. Here are some examples of sticks, branches, and logs of self-care from my own life – please keep in mind that these may look different for you:

- ☐ Sticks – eating regularly, bi-weekly grocery shopping, sleep

- ☐ Branches – yoga classes, therapy, meeting friends

- ☐ Logs – time off work, yoga retreats, holidays

To light a fire, we need lots of little sticks, but not as many branches or logs – the same can be said for self-care, unless you are going through a tumultuous time and need to take extra good care of yourself. If your version of self-care is mostly made up of logs, that will not be enough for your long-term health and well-being. One of my past clients shared with me how even after a two-week holiday, he felt completely exhausted. He was making time for logs of self-care, but the little sticks and branches of self-care were practically non-existent in his life. He felt overworked, under-appreciated, and had no time to look after himself, except for taking a two-week holiday twice a year. Remember, putting a log onto a dwindling fire will not make that fire any stronger – the sticks and branches are non-negotiable. Some pretty big changes were required in his life to make time for smaller, more regular items of self-care. Once he started to see the benefits of making time for these, it became easier to implement and maintain. It became non-negotiable. Not only did he start to feel better within himself, but he also became a better husband, father, friend, and employee. Having a self-care practice is powerful — I have seen this in my own life and in those of my clients.

When we think of our self-care practice as being composed of these sticks, branches, and logs, it makes it easier to maintain when life becomes challenging or overwhelming. For example, when I was finishing up my latest degree, I needed to prioritize making time to submit my assignments before the deadline (anyone who has completed a thesis will understand the sheer pain of this). This meant that I wasn't seeing friends as often or going to as many yoga classes, two really important self-care items for me. However, as long as I could maintain my sticks of self-care, such as regular meals and sleep, I could make it through the stressful period. Life is not perfect, and there will come times of stress for every one of us when we do not have the time, energy, or space in our lives for all the elements of self-care. If you have an unattainable self-care routine that isn't flexible and adaptable (remember that all-or-nothing thinking we want to leave behind), you'll soon find that your self-care practice is another source of stress, another thing on your to-do list — something we do not want to happen. In those times of overwhelm, ask yourself, 'What stick of self-care could I make time for today?'

The Self-Care List

Below is a list of different self-care activities to help inspire you to develop your own self-care practice. This list is not exhaustive — self-care can look different for all of us, so I encourage you to explore what fills your cup and makes you feel good. I highly recommend you pull out a pen and piece of paper and begin writing down what your sticks, branches, and logs of self-care might look like. This may change as time goes on, and that's OK.

- ☐ Therapy
- ☐ Eating regular meals
- ☐ Listening to music
- ☐ Reading
- ☐ Meeting friends
- ☐ Buying yourself flowers
- ☐ Having a bath
- ☐ Setting boundaries
- ☐ Going for a massage
- ☐ Wearing comfortable clothes
- ☐ Drinking enough water
- ☐ Stocking your house with food
- ☐ Spending time alone
- ☐ Lighting a nice candle
- ☐ Meditation
- ☐ Yoga
- ☐ Joyful movement

- ☐ Journalling
- ☐ Spending time in nature
- ☐ Skincare routine
- ☐ Taking a nap
- ☐ Saying no
- ☐ Hugs (from yourself or others)
- ☐ Self-pleasure practices
- ☐ Taking breaks
- ☐ Taking a holiday
- ☐ Lighting incense
- ☐ Making your bed
- ☐ Doing your laundry
- ☐ Cleaning the house
- ☐ Positive self-talk
- ☐ Affirmations or mantras
- ☐ Setting boundaries

Being Your Own Parent

Lately, I've seen a trend arise around self-care that paints it as always being fun and pleasurable. Self-care is certainly not always fun, and there will be times when you don't want to engage in whatever self-care practice you have deemed important for your long-term health and well-being. One of my clients told me recently that self-care confuses him and that he felt like self-care was all about 'being nice to yourself'. You could see how he thinks this — maybe this is how you feel about self-care too — when self-care is sold to us as having bubble baths, going for pints with the lads, or just general 'treat yo'self' vibes. This was when I introduced him to the concept of 'being your own parent'. Self-care is not always beautiful, and you may not want to practise it sometimes. Think about when you were a small child and wanted to go outside to play with your friends. You're so excited about having fun that you don't want to waste time putting on your shoes, socks, jacket, hat, and scarf. But it's freezing outside, so your mam or dad stops you and makes you do it before you leave. You're annoyed at them. To your childhood self, this feels like wasting time you could spend playing with your friends and having fun. Your parents know that not wrapping up will mean you develop a cold in a few days and won't be able to play with your friends at all. So they make you do it. Was it fun? No. Was it necessary for your health and well-being? Yes.

When we grow up and become adults, we no longer have a parent looking after our long-term health and well-being. We need to do that for ourselves. Self-care is not just about being nice to yourself (although it can sometimes be). It's also about being your own parent. The following table illustrates some comparisons between being nice to yourself and being your own parent:

Being Nice to Yourself	Being Your Own Parent
Treating yourself to a shopping trip because you've earned it	Looking at your financials and deciding to park the shopping this month
Scrolling on social media for two hours because it feels good in the moment	Spending two hours making it to an exercise class because it will make you feel better later
Ordering takeaway for dinner multiple times a week	Scheduling time to do a grocery shop
Having a glass of wine because you're stressed	Making time for stress management — for example, meditation or yoga
Choosing fast food because it tastes good	Choosing a home-cooked, nutrient-rich meal because it tastes good *and* makes your body feel good

Can you see a pattern in the above comparisons? Being nice to yourself often involves prioritizing 'in the moment' pleasure. Being your own parent weighs up the pros and cons of your decisions, evaluates the consequences, and considers your future self before it makes one. Self-parenting requires you to act in ways that may not feel pleasurable in the moment but are in service of your future self. To truly look after yourself and your long-term health and well-being, you will need a healthy balance of being nice to yourself and self-parenting.

The Importance of Boundaries

'I would have considered myself a chocoholic; not any more. It's amazing to figure out why I often turned towards chocolate and other sugary foods.' These were the words spoken by a past client of mine who realized that a lack of healthy boundaries was feeding her 'addiction' to chocolate. Wild, right? She went on to share her experience with me:

> I enjoy the chocolate when I have it now, but I don't need it like I used to. I feel very neutral about it. I used to think people were crazy when they said they look at chocolate and an apple in the same way, and now I do the same. I'm one of those people I used to roll my eyes at. I can't believe it! Intuitive eating has saved me.

For this person, a lack of healthy boundaries resulted in her feeling tired, exhausted, and resentful, which led to overeating chocolate and other sugary foods. Chocolate gave her a burst of energy, but not the kind she really needed. Food was not the correct solution to her needs — it was like putting a plaster over a wound that needed a stitch. Until she implemented the boundaries required in her life, the low energy and 'chocolate addiction' ensued. Once the appropriate boundaries were implemented, she found herself feeling calmer and more at peace around food, along with an overall feeling of contentment about her life. The difference that a few small boundaries made was incredible.

A lack of healthy boundaries is not something to be ashamed of — I see it come up incredibly often in my practice. Many people did not grow up in families where boundary setting was modelled or asking for your needs to be met was a common and acceptable practice. This is no one's fault; it's often passed down from generation to generation until someone in the line decides to change things. Your boundaries are a roadmap to getting your needs met. It includes more than just saying no and involves openly communicating your feelings and asking for what you need. Boundaries are not a way of getting back at anyone or a way to cause arguments or ruptures in your relationships with others — quite the opposite. They protect your relationships and allow them to grow and thrive. How could someone possibly show up for you in the way you need if you do not tell them and vice versa? Some people may not be able to meet your boundaries, but if you constantly abandon them to please others, it will eventually affect the relationship, not to mention your health, as demonstrated in the above example. A lack of healthy boundaries can affect your relationship with food in a negative way since food can be used to fill the void. This is why I often see in clinic a correlation between a lack of healthy boundaries and an unhealthy relationship with food.

Boundaries can be set in a very loving way — this will all come down to your communication skills, which take time and practice to develop. Setting limits with others or asking for your needs to be met can feel very uncomfortable, especially if it's new for you. If this is a new skill you are developing, you may be met with some resistance to your boundaries from others.

This is normal and expected. Reinforcing your boundaries by holding people accountable is part of the process, despite the discomfort that may arise. Their resistance is not a sign that you should back down and abandon your boundaries.

So how do you figure out if a boundary needs to be set? A question I ask myself when I have a sneaky suspicion that I need to implement or reinforce a boundary is:

> If I say yes to this person/project/activity/behaviour, am I saying no to myself?

This will very quickly help you understand your next step and whether you need to set or reinforce a boundary. The first step is knowing. The second is to take action.

This brings us to boundary setting itself — how do we communicate our boundaries to others? This will require you to be highly connected to yourself, to be self-aware and understand your emotions. How could you express your feelings to someone else if you do not understand them yourself first? I hope this explains why working through parts 1 and 2 of the book was essential to understanding Part 3. When you are reconnected to yourself, understand your emotions, and feel ready to set a boundary, there is an accessible template you can use:

> 'I feel _____ when you _____, and what I need is _____.'

Your boundaries are unique to you, so there are a million examples I could use to demonstrate what this might look like. Since the topic of this book is to rebuild your relationship with food and body image, I will use an example that comes up very often in my clinic relating to this topic: setting a boundary with someone who comments on your body or food choices. Using the template above, this could sound something like:

'I feel judged when you comment on my body or food choices, and what I need is for you to refrain from commenting on either of these in the future.'

To add a loving edge to this boundary, you could follow it with:

'I understand you may not be aware of this, but I am communicating it with you because I care about you and our relationship and want to continue connecting with you.'

This small section on boundary-setting only scratches the surface of this topic. There are entire books written about boundary setting, and for good reason — a lack of boundaries can cause many problems in life — but also because setting limits with others is hard work. This is partly because we all fear rejection, some of us more than others, depending on how asking for our needs to be met was responded to in our childhood. As the saying goes, 'People who mind don't matter and people who matter don't mind.' Trust that by setting boundaries you are doing right by yourself, but you are also doing right by the relationship. This is one of the greatest gifts of self-care you can give yourself. You're worth it and your needs matter just as much as anyone else's.

The Importance of Rest

Is taking time to rest easy or difficult for you? For many people I work with, it's the latter. The inspiration for this section came to me while lying on a sunlounger beside a pool in Portugal. How ironic. Making time for rest and switching off from work is difficult for me, just like it is for my clients. Not so much in the 'answering your emails' way, but in the sense that there are always new ideas running around my head, waiting to be born. I get my best ideas when I'm taking time to relax, hence the inspiration for this section came to me while resting. The same happens when I'm on a massage table, reading a book, or sitting out on the balcony with a cup of tea. This is not a coincidence. Creating space for rest is key to unlocking your creativity. I have to make a conscious effort to switch off, and I'm not always successful, but I continue to try. The attempt to rest and the acknowledgement of its importance is key. When we slow down and rest, we create space. Space to think, to feel, and to reflect on what is within. Creating this space in your life can unlock insights about yourself that you were previously unaware of. Rest should not be underestimated.

Where are you on your own to-do list? Not considering rest as part of this to-do list can have some serious consequences. I have had a few clients in the past where a lack of rest was the primary cause of their issues with food, mainly in the case of binge eating, overeating, or emotional eating. Looking after yourself is imperative so you can show up for not just yourself but for others in your life too. Rest is an essential part of looking after yourself. Taking the time to rest allows your nervous system to rebalance, and relaxation is key to long-term health and vitality. You are your most valuable asset. The possibility of thriving for a long time is within reach, but only if you put your health before all else.

When I speak about making time for rest with my clients it's not uncommon for them to say that this feels selfish to them, or that they feel guilt when purposely taking time to rest. Hustle culture is mainly to blame for this. We have been taught to prioritize doing over being. Doing is rewarded. Being is not. This societal belief system feeds into what we value in ourselves and others and impacts our behaviour and how we show up in our everyday lives. But you do not have to abide by these faulty societal beliefs. You can begin to create a new path for yourself by exploring the value that self-care and rest brings to your life.

Affirmations

Today, I will take one step towards greater self-care.

I prioritize my own needs.

Boundaries protect my own well-being and that of my relationships.

It is safe for me to rest.

I care for myself with love, as I would for another.

Taking care of myself is my first responsibility.

Chapter 12:

Stress Management

On a scale of zero to ten, with zero being having no stress and ten being extremely stressed, how would you rate your current stress level? Don't overthink your answer. Even if you feel you 'shouldn't' feel stressed, or if you think the number you gravitate towards doesn't match the circumstances of what you expect should cause this level of stress, if a high number feels true for you, then that's your truth. We all have different-sized stress buckets – I could have a small stress bucket, and you could have a large one or vice versa. Once this bucket starts to overflow, you will suffer the consequences of mismanaged stress levels.

As I write this, I'm just a few weeks out from delivering the first completed draft of this book you are holding in your hands, so I'd say my stress level is a solid eight – LOL, how ironic! I'm always real with my clients, which is why I'm being real with you in this book. Experiencing stress in real life, alongside my professional experience, helps me to help you, the reader, and all of my clients to manage their stress. I'm human.

I get stressed, too, and I know how difficult it can be to manage. I don't always get it right and I'm far from perfect, but that's not the point. We will all react in ways we'd rather not when we look back in hindsight and realize that stress got in the way. Awareness is the key to learning, growing, and better handling your stress levels. Right now, I know that my stress level will drop once I've delivered my manuscript. This is temporary stress; it will pass. Stress is not always a bad thing — it can help us reach our goals or get shit done.

The problems arise when elevated levels of stress are chronic and not acute. If stress goes unchecked or unmanaged, it can wreak havoc on our health. Managing your stress levels is one of the most underrated changes you can make on any health and wellness journey. It might not be as sexy as green smoothies or matcha lattes, but it's crucial for long-term health and well-being. Stress is like a silent destroyer. And if you let that destroyer roam free in your mind and body without putting some boundaries around it, it will cause severe damage. I speak about stress so often in my practice because without taking a deep look at the stress in your life and developing some stress management skills it's impossible to truly look after yourself and work on improving your health. It's essential, not optional.

We cannot avoid stress — as I say to my clients, 'Life throws shit at us all the time,' but how you respond to and manage that stress is the key. None of us has any idea what shit life will throw at us, but if we develop some vital stress management skills, we can rest assured that we can handle whatever comes our way. Learning how to manage stress is a lifelong practice, but one that will contribute to a happy, healthy, and purposeful life.

What Is Stress?

Stress is a feeling of emotional or physical tension that can arise from any stress-causing factor or 'stressor'. The combination of reactions to stress is also known as the 'fight or flight' response, due to its evolution as a survival mechanism to enable mammals to escape life-threatening situations. We can thank this response for allowing our ancestors to survive and pass on their genetic heritage to us. The stress response is a vital and primitive component for maintaining life. However, in today's world, the stress response is turned on more often than the body and mind would like. During this stress response, the nervous system is activated, and specific hormones such as adrenaline and cortisol are released, which increase blood pressure, heart rate, and muscular tension. Energy is diverted away from bodily systems seen as less important, such as the digestive, reproductive, and immune systems.

Stress is not definitively destructive, and pressure can be helpful for performance during brief periods of stress. However, the stress response can become more damaging than the stressor itself when it becomes chronic and mismanaged, leading to ill health. Balancing tensions is key to ensuring that the stress response does not wreak havoc on the body's systems and contribute to illness. Too little stress and we become bored and dissatisfied. Too much stress and we can burn out and suffer from illnesses like depression and anxiety. Negative stress occurs when you perceive the challenge or situation you encounter as difficult, painful, or dangerous — for example, the death of a loved one, an unrelenting work schedule, or a divorce. Positive stress comes from doing something challenging for the first time, the physical challenge of a good workout, moving to a new home, or starting a new job.

We experience stress from three main sources:

1. Physical: physical stress arises from illness, lack of exercise, poor nutrition, inadequate sleep, ageing, and the life cycle, such as during adolescence or menopause. We may also experience physical stress as a physiological response to environmental and mental stress, in the form of aching muscles, headaches, nausea, and anxiety.

2. Environmental: environmental stress comes from outside of yourself. It may be in the form of the weather, noise, traffic, or air pollution. It could also come from work, home, or relationships — for example, work deadlines, presentations, competing priorities, job interviews, relationship problems, financial problems, or the loss of loved ones.

3. Mental: mental stress comes from inside of yourself, primarily your thoughts. The brain cannot distinguish between fact and fiction. Any problem, real or imaginary, can trigger the stress response. This means that even if it's not really happening, but you're imagining it happening in the mind, the reaction in the body is the same. Interpretation is the key. For example, interpreting a friend's lack

of response to a phone call as them not wanting to be your friend any more is bound to be stressful. Interpreting it as a preoccupation with themselves and their own life won't be as triggering.

Chronic stress occurs when stressors are unrelenting — for example, during a messy divorce, a chronic illness, caring for a loved one, or long-term financial worries. It may also occur when small stressors accumulate and you struggle to recover from any of them. During times of chronic stress, when the fight or flight response goes unchecked, the adrenal glands secrete corticoids (adrenaline or epinephrine and norepinephrine), which inhibit digestion, reproduction, growth, tissue repair, and the responses of the immune and inflammatory systems. In other words, some very important functions that keep the body healthy begin to shut down. Fortunately, the 'relaxation response' can turn the stress response off and therefore protect the functionality and vitality of the mind and body.[1]

The Autonomic Nervous System

The autonomic nervous system (ANS) regulates the body's internal states and plays a direct role in the physical response to stress. It operates unconsciously, meaning that you do not have to consciously direct its functioning. For example, you do not have to ask your heart to beat or your lungs to breathe — it does this for you without direction. The ANS is made up of two different groups of nerves: the sympathetic nerves and the parasympathetic nerves. These subsystems of the ANS, the sympathetic nervous system (SNS) and the parasympathetic nervous system (PNS), have opposite functions.

For example, the SNS may prepare an organism for a flight or fight response by increasing the heart rate, breathing rate, muscle tension, metabolism and blood pressure, along with dilating the pupils and diverting blood from the skin to the skeletal muscles. Blood is directed away from the extremities and digestive system, leading to the hands and feet becoming cold or clammy.[1] It also causes the adrenal glands to release adrenaline and noradrenaline, helping the body prepare for potential or sudden energy output. In short, it acts to mobilize the body's resources in response to an emergency or a stressful situation.[2] These stressful situations can be either real or imaginary – both can cause the cerebral cortex in the brain to send a signal to the hypothalamus, which then stimulates the SNS to make a series of changes in the body.

On the other hand, the PNS, otherwise known as the 'rest and digest' nervous system, reverses or normalizes the effects of the SNS and generally acts to save energy or maintain resting body function.[2] The nerves of the PNS enter the body at the top and bottom of the spine and help to slow the stress response and repair the body. It stimulates the relaxation response and functions mainly during normal and non-stressful conditions.[2] Therefore, this system is most active when the body is at rest, where the PNS is focused on controlling the digestive system and conserving body energy.

Although the SNS and PNS are often regarded as having opposite effects, the two systems generally work together to control the function of a given organ.[2] The relaxation response can be turned on once you decide that a situation is no longer dangerous. When this happens, the brain stops sending emergency signals to your brain stem, resulting in a cessation of panic messages sent to the nervous system. It takes three minutes after these mechanisms are switched off for the fight-or-flight response to burn out. As a result, the metabolism, heart rate, breathing rate, muscle tension, and blood pressure all return to normal levels.[1]

When explaining the nervous system in clinic, I think of its two branches as the 'red zone' (SNS) and the 'green zone' (PNS). In an ideal world, we would spend most of our time in the green zone and dip in and out of the red zone when we need to or when danger hits. That danger could be an actual dangerous situation, such as a near-collision on the motorway, or it could be in the form of an upcoming work deadline. As I have explained above, the stress response is vital for survival, and when we utilize it for short bursts of energy it can be incredibly useful. However, we run into problems when we stay in the red zone for prolonged periods and do not learn how to down-regulate into the green zone. Nervous system regulation hinges on your ability to recognize when you find yourself in the red zone and then relies upon appropriate strategies to help you return to the green zone. In essence, nervous system regulation will require you to learn how to calm and rebalance the nervous system.

I spent two years learning about the physiological stress response when I studied counselling and psychotherapy. It was one of the most fascinating learning experiences I've ever had, both personally and professionally, and it's heavily influenced my practice and how I live my own life. I'll never forget one day in particular, when my stress response trainer, Ray McKiernan, demonstrated the stress response to us in class. He handed one of my classmates a galvanic skin resistance machine that monitors small changes in the skin's electrical resistance, a physiochemical response to emotional arousal that increases during SNS activity. He asked her to place her thumb and index finger on the device and then work on calming her nervous system. We had spent over a year practising this individually, so we could (almost) do it on demand. She closed her eyes and began to breathe very slowly and deeply, since utilizing the breath is one of the most powerful ways to consciously regulate the nervous system. The results were shown on a tablet, demonstrating her stress response through a graphical representation.

As she began to breathe and calm her nervous system, the lines on the corresponding graph flattened out. Then he said to her, 'I'm going to ask you a question.' The lines became more erratic. Even though no question had been posed, the antici-pation and uncertainty of what was coming were enough to trigger the stress response. Remember, the stress response occurs from both real and imaginary danger. He then asked her to calm her nervous system again, and the lines flattened out. Then he said, 'Imagine someone you dislike has just entered the room.' Once again, the line graph instantly changed and became more erratic. Ray continued, 'Now imagine they're standing right in front of you.' You know where I'm going with this — the graph became even more erratic. For the final time, he asked her to calm her nervous system, and the lines flat-tened once more. We witnessed a visible activation of the SNS and the subsequent activation of the PNS or relaxation response. It was incredible to watch and really showed the importance of having the skills to down-regulate the nervous system. How many of us walk around with consistent SNS activation, unknowingly living life in the red zone?

To regulate your nervous system, you must first notice how stress shows up in your body. Only then can you begin to put strategies in place to manage it.

How Do You Cope with Stress?

Before trying to change how you manage your stress, you must first understand how you currently cope with it. Listed below are some common ways of coping with stressful events:

- ☐ I ignore my own needs and just work harder.

- ☐ I turn to my friends for support.

- ☐ I eat to self-soothe.

- ☐ I exercise.

- ☐ I get frustrated and irritable.

- ☐ I take a break to relax.

- ☐ I smoke a cigarette.

- ☐ I drink more alcohol than usual.

- ☐ I withdraw emotionally.

- ☐ I maintain a healthy diet.

- ☐ I ignore the source of my stress and hope it will stop bothering me.

☐ I tackle the source of my stress head on, and focus on what I can control.

☐ I worry about the problem and how I will deal with it.

This is not an exhaustive list: there are all sorts of ways people deal with stress, and it would be impossible to write down all of them! There are lots of amazing resources available to help develop better stress management skills. One of these is *The Relaxation and Stress Reduction Workbook*, which has lots of exercises to help you gain more insight into how you deal with stress. It can be difficult to pinpoint exactly how stress impacts your life, so these kinds of workbooks are really useful to slowly work through your existing coping mechanisms and learn to develop new, healthy habits.[1]

Noticing Your Stress

How can you begin managing your stress levels if you cannot recognize them in the first place? By tuning into your stress now, you reduce the risk of stress affecting your health in the future. Stress can show up in several different ways in your body, mind, and behaviour. We all feel stress differently — how it manifests for me may be different to how it does for you. What happens when you feel stressed? Are you aware of any changes that occur when you feel stressed, or can you notice when your stress levels begin to rise? If not, don't worry, but it's worthwhile to spend some time and energy getting to know your individual stress response on a deeper level.

Although the way each of us feels stress differs, there are some signs to watch out for. The below table describes several ways that stress can show up, physically, emotionally, and behaviourally. This will give you some signs and symptoms to be aware of, but completing a stress diary (see the next section) is the best way to get a deeper understanding of your own stress symptoms:

Physical	Emotional	Behavioural
Muscle tension	Unusually irritable or angry	Eating more or less
Nausea	Anxious or nervous	Sleeping more or less
Shallow or erratic breathing	Irrational fears	Working much harder
Indigestion	Lack of self-confidence	Working much less
IBS symptoms	Feeling inadequate	Losing interest in sex
Diarrhoea or constipation	Aggressiveness	Nail-biting
Headaches or migraines	Tiredness, apathy, lack of energy	Talking more or less
Dry mouth	Difficulty making simple decisions	Drinking or smoking more
Difficulty sleeping	Being unable to concentrate	Licking your lips frequently

Keeping a Stress Diary

When I start working on managing stress with my clients, I always recommend they begin the process by keeping a stress diary. I did this as part of my counselling training and it helped highlight the stressors in my life, such as the things that triggered my stress response. Suddenly, I could see patterns contributing to daily stress, which made me question the impact of certain situations I found myself in and the decisions I was making. A word of warning: once you see this for yourself, you can't unsee it. If you want to change your life, it will require you to confront some difficult things about yourself. It can be uncomfortable, but awareness is the first step to change. Without it, nothing changes. So although it may be difficult to look at your life in this way or come face to face with how you react to stressors, it's necessary. If you commit to keeping a stress diary for some time, I promise it will lead you to important insights that will help you to manage your stress levels.

I usually suggest putting a timeline on how long you plan to keep a stress diary. This can help you to actually start. Think about it — how would you feel if I asked you to keep a stress diary for two weeks versus if I asked you to keep one indefinitely? The former usually feels more manageable for most people. You might decide to continue with your stress diary after the initial two weeks, which would be excellent, but let's set a two-week timeline for now. For two weeks, I invite you to document your response anytime you come up against a stressor. You can do this in a fancy journal, the notes function on your phone, a Word document, or a simple notebook from your local shop — whatever works.

Here is an example of a stress diary entry, with prompts you can use to identify stressors and the corresponding reactions:

Time: 2 p.m.

Stressful event: colleague was rude

Symptoms: anger, tightness in stomach, feeling hot, overthinking

Stress level from 0–10: 5

As you can see, it's pretty straightforward but will require you to check in with your inner landscape and explore what is going on. If you're struggling with reconnecting with your inner wisdom, I recommend going back and rereading Chapter 5 to help you with this.

Managing Your Stress

Managing your stress levels requires you to first notice when you are in your red zone and then employ an appropriate strategy to bring yourself back down into the green zone. There are, therefore, two steps to this process:

Step 1: notice your symptoms of stress

Step 2: employ a stress management strategy

The second step will require you to develop stress management skills that let the body know you are now safe and that the danger which triggered the stress response has passed. These stress management skills activate the relaxation response, allowing the body to calm down, as illustrated in the diagram below.

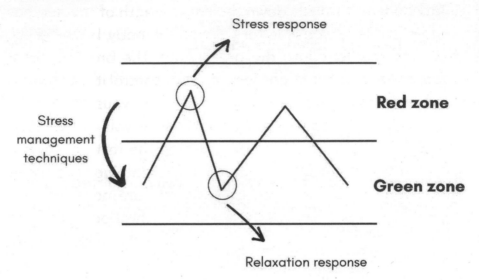

To employ an effective stress management strategy that will initiate the relaxation response during moments of SNS activation, you will need to develop some techniques to help you wind down. The number of relaxation techniques available is endless – I could fill a book on this topic alone – but I will describe a few of my favourites here. You will most likely need to play around with different techniques to find out what works best for you.

Breathing techniques
How you breathe has a direct impact on how you feel. As we have discussed, the ANS operates unconsciously, meaning that we cannot consciously control it. However, we can

consciously control the breath, and since the breath stimulates the vagus nerve, which regulates the stress response by activating the relaxation response, it has a direct impact on the nervous system. The vagus nerve is the longest cranial nerve in the body – it travels down the entire length of the nervous system and is responsible for calming the body, bringing you from the red zone into the green zone. The breath is your superpower, and if you can learn how to control it, you access the power to control the state of your nervous system. By breathing slowly and deeply into the belly, you can turn off the fight-or-flight response and turn on the rest-and-digest or relaxation response. In yoga, we call breathing techniques 'pranayama' or 'breath work', of which there are many different types, but these go beyond the scope of this book. Let's just keep it really simple for now by learning the yogic breath. Here's how to practise it:

1. Lie down on your back and close your eyes.

2. Place both hands on your belly.

3. Begin to breathe deeply through the nose into the belly, breathing into the hands and filling out the belly like a balloon.

4. Feel the belly rise on the inhale and fall on the exhale.

5. Expand the breath to the ribs and chest, imagining that you are filling three different compartments with breath as you inhale: the belly, the ribs, and the upper chest.

6. On the exhale, feel the breath empty from the chest, the ribs and finally, the belly.

7. Slow the breath down with every breath cycle, making each inhale and exhale slower and deeper than the last.

8. Lengthen the exhale, making each exhale longer than the inhale.

9. Repeat at least ten times.

10. Allow your breath to settle back to your natural breath. Notice how you feel.

The most fantastic thing about deep breathing is that it can be done anywhere, and no one would notice a thing. The steps above can be adjusted to fit the situation. For example, you might not always be able to close your eyes and lie down on your back. This isn't necessary to practise deep breathing. It doesn't need to be scheduled. You can use it before that big presentation at work, when you're trying to calm yourself down at home before responding to your family, or in the car when you're stuck in rush-hour traffic. So simple but so powerful.

Yoga

Anyone who knows me will know that yoga is my jam. I am a yoga teacher but I'm also an avid student, and when I'm feeling stressed, there is no better tonic for me than to head to a yoga class. There are many yoga styles: some work better for calming the nervous system than others, particularly slow and gentle forms of yoga, such as yin and restorative yoga. That's not to say that you won't discover some relaxation benefits from a faster, more active class — I certainly do — but the intention is different. When I go to a yin or restorative yoga class, my intention is purely to rest, recuperate, and take care of my nervous system so that it can take care of me — building strength and stamina is not the goal.

Yoga nidra

> '*Yoga Nidra is a state of complete bodily relaxation, in which the mind rests in a suspended state awake, yet calm, and free of all distractions. The body, senses and material mind are magnetized.*'
> — Shri Brahmananda Sarasvati

For those of you who have attended a yoga class, yoga nidra is sometimes practised in the last ten minutes, in what is often called 'shavasana'. However, yoga nidra, also known as yogic sleep, is a practice in itself that guides you to complete bodily relaxation. When practising yoga nidra, you will be instructed to lie down on your back, get comfortable, and close your eyes, and a teacher will guide you through it. The instructions will include tuning into the mind and body through techniques such as rotation of consciousness, visualization, breathing, and awareness of bodily sensations. Yoga nidra is a fascinating practice that allows you to relax the mind by relaxing the body, and like other techniques I mention here, there are entire books written on the subject, such as *Yoga Nidra* by Swami Satyananda Saraswati. Saraswati describes yoga nidra as a state between wakefulness and dreaming, which creates an inner awareness and enables us to connect with the unconscious mind. It allows us to leave the waking state and move into the deep sleep state, yet remain fully awake. Yoga nidra has many benefits, including freeing the mind of unnecessary and negative thoughts, providing the overactive mind with a rest, promoting calmness and relieving stress, along with the physical benefits of relaxing the muscles in the body. It is such a simple practice that it can be practised universally and is suitable for everyone, no matter their age or state of health.

Exercise or movement
Exercise or movement helps manage stress levels because it reduces stress hormones, such as adrenaline and cortisol, and stimulates the production of endorphins, or feel-good hormones. When you begin building a regular and consistent exercise routine, it's important that you engage with a form of movement that you enjoy — one that doesn't feel like torture (we've all been there). We will speak about this more in Chapter 14.

Progressive muscle relaxation
Progressive muscle relaxation helps you recognize the difference between tension and relaxation in each major muscle group in the body. We all carry tension in the body from the everyday stresses of life, and we often don't even realize it. By bringing your attention to what a tense vs a relaxed muscle feels like, you can consciously release any locked-in tension in the body and identify it in the future. For example, right now,

while you read this, I invite you to bring your attention to your jaw. Are you holding it tightly, or can you feel any tension in the area? If so, release it by parting the lips ever so slightly. This is essentially how we practise progressive muscle relaxation, but we do it throughout the whole body in a practice that usually takes 15–20 minutes. You can download an audio version of this from my website, nutritionwithniamh.com.

Meditation
Meditation is thousands of years old, and as a practice, it involves using techniques to focus and observe the mind. In doing so, peace of mind is created, alongside other benefits such as improved focus and concentration, mental clarity, and self-awareness. Although one of the goals is to settle the mind, meditation is not about clearing the mind of all thoughts but observing them without judgement. I like to think that we all have an inner landscape with its own ever-changing weather system, and meditation allows us to take ourselves out of the tornado of our thoughts and observe this inner landscape from a bird's-eye view. You will find lots of free meditations online, or my personal favourite place to meditate is through the Headspace app.

*

I encourage you to try some of the above techniques, either on your own or through online resources or by finding yoga studios in your area that may provide them. Building some of these relaxation techniques into your life will substantially impact your stress levels and how you manage them.

Taking a Stress Inventory

Many things in life may cause you stress. Unfortunately, some of these are unavoidable and out of your control. Developing effective stress management skills is vital to prepare yourself for these eventualities. But some situations are within your control. If you really want to get serious about reducing the amount of stress in your life, you will need to evaluate whether or not you're ready to remove, or at least reduce, the number of controllable stressors in your day-to-day.

For example, suppose you have a difficult relationship with a friend or family member. They might make you feel stressed when you are around them, or they may demand a lot from you, more than you can currently give. You cannot change the other person. You cannot make them act in a way that makes you feel less stressed when you are around them. However, you can set boundaries with this person that protect your well-being and the future of the relationship.

Below are some examples of potentially controllable stressors. This is just a general overview — your own lived experience and circumstances will also play a role in the examples. I am not suggesting that it is easy to change some of these stressors — quite the opposite — but to transform your life, you may need to make some challenging choices. Transformation is never easy, but it's always worth it. If you identify with some of these stressors and feel stuck as to how you should proceed, I highly recommend reaching out to a professional, such as a therapist, to help you move forward and examine your life on a deeper level:

☐ Unhappy in your job

☐ Working long hours

☐ Relationship problems

☐ A heavy workload or too much responsibility

☐ Emotional problems (depression, anxiety, low self-esteem and so on)

☐ A lack of personal or professional boundaries

☐ Fear and uncertainty

☐ Unrealistic expectations

☐ Resistance to change

Keeping a stress diary will also give you an insight into the situations causing stress. Once you have identified these, you can evaluate whether or not they are within your control and if there is something you could do to improve the situation — be honest with yourself. A therapist could also help you with this.

The STOP Technique

I love a good acronym, and this one will really help you when you come up against stressful situations. In these moments of stress, having an easy-to-access, step-by-step technique can be very powerful. The STOP technique will remind you to check in with yourself, so that you can evaluate your response before responding:

S: Stop
Very simply, stop before you react. When you carve out some space between urge and action, you can better evaluate your response before you respond:

T: Take a breath
Take a deep, slow breath into the belly, followed by a long, slow exhale. This may be difficult during times of stress, but making the time to do this, even for a few seconds, will help to calm the nervous system so that you can respond from a calm, rather than an activated, nervous system.

O: Observe
Observe what's going on within. Are you having a stress response in your body? Are you experiencing any physical sensations of stress? Is something being triggered for you? Is this really about you or the other person or situation?

P: Proceed
Only when you've walked yourself through the above steps should you proceed with a response. Can you respond, rather than react? What response would your future self thank you for? Have you come up against a similar situation in the past that could guide your response? Do you need to employ an effective stress management technique, either in the moment or at the first opportunity? Utilizing the STOP technique will help you to manage your

stress levels on a moment-to-moment basis, leading to feelings of balance and contentment and, therefore, better health for the long-term.

Affirmations

I inhale peace, I exhale stress.

I can handle anything that comes my way today.

I focus on what I can control and let go of what I cannot.

I am working on managing my stress.

I breathe slowly and deeply.

I have the power to make positive changes in my life.

Chapter 13:

Food and Nutrition

'Oh, you're a nutritionist? I suppose you never eat anything bad then, do you?'

I cannot count how many times I've heard this over the years. Announcing I'm a nutritionist at a table of people I've never met before always leads to an interesting conversation that shows how much diet culture has infiltrated our attitudes and perceptions around food. I love chocolate, cake, and pizza just as much as the next person, but I remember feeling like a 'bad' nutritionist at the start of my career because of this — hello, diet culture! Once people get to know me, they quickly discover that restrictions and rules around food are not my jam and that dietary perfection is not necessary to be healthy. When we think about food and nutrition, it's often in these black-and-white terms because of the impact that diet culture has had on us all. It has morphed our perceptions of what is required to be healthy and looks at nutrition in reductionist terms. In fact, when recently asked, 'So what do you think is the one food that's causing most of our health issues? Probably sugar, right?' I responded with, 'I think our mindset around food and health is what's actually causing most of the problems.'

It might surprise you to hear that these days I actually talk very little about nutrition on a daily basis with my clients. That's because, for most people, more information is not what's needed to improve their eating habits. A connection to their own inner wisdom is. Nutrition is powerful and it can have a substantial impact on your health, but only if a healthy relationship with food is in place. I'm sure you all know what you 'should' eat, right? We have so much information at our fingertips, yet many people still struggle with their diet. Believe it or not, eating well becomes much easier when you are connected to your inner expert and are in tune with what does and does not feel good in your body. That's why a huge part of this book is dedicated to the 'reconnect' stage of the process and why this needs to come before implementing any changes around what you eat. Nonetheless, if you are ready to dive into the topic of food and nutrition, I have some easy-to-follow guidelines to share with you. Nutrition is a huge topic in itself, one that couldn't possibly be covered in one chapter, so I will mention some essentials to get you started. If you only follow the guidelines I suggest in the next few pages, you will begin to see improvements in your general health and well-being over time.

Gentle Nutrition: A New Way of Thinking

Eating for general health and well-being doesn't need to be complicated, and in this chapter I aim to uncomplicate it.

You may have heard some of this information before, but it often gets glossed over in favour of rigid, inflexible, sensational, or scaremongering-type headlines. I hate to break it to you, but there is no secret, no silver bullet regarding food and nutrition. If someone tells you that their plan or way of eating is the answer to all your problems, run. We are all different and therefore have different lifestyles, nutritional needs, likes and dislikes, and preparation skills. Not taking these into account is a recipe for disaster. Cookie-cutter diet plans do not work. Getting the basics right is critical, and if this is all you do, consistently, over time, you will begin to see changes in how you feel. Food is very powerful, and it can have a massive impact on how you feel in your body on a daily basis, so it should not be underestimated. However, as we have covered already, food isn't the only thing that impacts your health and it needs to slot into a holistic set of strategies.

Let me introduce you to the concept of gentle nutrition. Unlike mainstream nutrition rhetoric peddled by diet culture, gentle nutrition is about self-care, not self-control. It's about looking after your body and using food to nourish you in a positive way that makes you feel good on the inside rather than using it to control what you look like on the outside. In the words of Rachael Hartley, author of *Gentle Nutrition*, 'gentle nutrition is a flexible, non-diet, and evidence-based approach to healthy eating, one that centers on you and your unique individual needs'.[1] Doing this will require a deep connection to what is within because only you know what does and doesn't feel good in your body. Gentle nutrition is about dropping the rigidity around food and embracing flexibility and imperfection. It is the last principle of intuitive eating for a reason. If it's targeted first, it's usually approached with a 'rule' or diet mindset. When you apply the initial stages of the intuitive eating approach and learn how to reconnect with your inner expert, you will find yourself embracing and accepting nutritional concepts in a more free-flowing way that enriches your life rather than taking from it. Healthy eating is all about having a healthy balance of foods and a healthy relationship with food. We can't have one without the other. We need to make food choices that honour our health and our taste buds while making us feel well.

You don't have to eat a perfect diet to be healthy, so let's drop that idea right now. All foods have a place. If you were to eat 'bad' food 24/7, I could guarantee you that your body would respond by craving an apple or some eggs on toast. Likewise, cravings will be hard to ignore if you never eat 'bad' foods. It's what you eat consistently over time that matters – progress, not perfection.

The Foundations of Gentle Nutrition

A range of foundational concepts makes up the basis of gentle nutrition. Keeping these in mind as you begin to consider food and nutrition will help you embrace this part of the journey with a gentle nutrition mindset, rather than one steeped in diet mentality.

Adequacy
The first and perhaps most important consideration is to ensure you are eating enough food. This is where diet culture has really affected our thinking and led us to believe that a

small quantity of food should be enough. The food that is recommended on some diet plans wouldn't be enough to sustain a toddler, let alone a fully grown adult. Only you know how much food you need in a day, since only you can check in with your hunger, fullness, and satisfaction cues. There are recommended energy intake guidelines in nutritional science, but these are only guidelines. The best guide you have to define how much food is needed is your own body. These needs may also change from day to day, depending on your activity level, among other factors. It's entirely normal for your hunger levels to vary — you could be starving one day and not the next. I encourage you to trust the body in these moments. Keep in mind that even if you feel like you are eating enough but are not eating regularly and your eating pattern is chaotic or you are going long periods without eating, this will also cause stress on the body. I see this most often in clients who eat very little during the day but eat a lot at night. A lack of food during the day will often catch up on you in the evening or in the following days. Try to eat regularly where possible, ideally every three to four hours (this is a guideline, not a rule).

Balance
You've probably heard 'eat a balanced diet' many times. Balance comes from eating enough carbohydrates, protein, and fat throughout the day, ideally at most meals. Restricting certain macronutrients creates nutritional gaps that are very hard to fill. There is no need to micromanage this, and counting macros is unnecessary. I will share more about how to do this when I speak about balancing your meals using the five funda-mentals formula.

Variety

A healthy diet contains a wide variety of foods and food groups. Diet plans tend to be very restrictive and may even advocate for removing certain foods or entire food groups. Unless this is for a specific medical reason or grounded in a clear why, these kinds of blanket recommendations are dodgy, sometimes even dangerous. Let's take dairy, for example. Dairy provides substantial amounts of protein and calcium in the diets of many. If it's removed, there is a potential risk of deficiency if it's not replaced with an appropriate substitute. Eating the same foods day in and day out could also lead to deficiencies. Try to mix it up by eating different flavours, textures, colours, cuisines, and types of food to get the most comprehensive array of nutrients possible.

Addition not subtraction

'Avoid foods high in saturated fat like butter, cream and red meat.'

'Cut back on salt.'

'Reduce foods high in fat and sugar.'

'Do not eat these foods every day.'

How do you feel when you read these statements? Do you feel free and at ease? Or do you feel panicky or concerned? Many clients are terrified when they come to me with a food or life-style-related issue since they fear I'm going to recommend they remove their favourite foods from their diet. Let's get one thing straight: I am not the food police, nor do I desire to be.

As we have established, the more intense the restriction, the more intense the craving, and, therefore, the more intense the overeating. Rather than advocating for 'reducing', 'removing', 'cutting back', or 'avoiding', I recommend adding in more foods that make your body feel well. Language is important, and this will help to prevent a scarcity response.

You can do this while being conscious of how certain foods affect your health, without applying rigid rules to their consumption. Technically, yes, there are some foods that you may benefit from 'cutting back on', but if you perceive these recommendations as rigid or inflexible, it can have the opposite effect. So, for example:

Rather than: don't use butter.

Embrace: be conscious of butter intake.

Rather than: cut back on red meat intake.

Embrace: be conscious of red meat intake.

We know that consuming a high quantity of red and processed meat can increase your risk of colorectal cancer.[2] You can take this information on board to inform your decisions around food without having to cut red and processed meat out entirely if it's something you enjoy eating as part of a balanced diet.

By adding in foods that make your body feel well, you will ultimately improve your health. You can consider this concept going into mealtimes by remembering to embrace 'nutrition addition'. Ask yourself, what can I add to this meal to boost the nutrition quality? Perhaps more fruit or vegetables, wholegrains, or nuts and seeds? This is something your health would benefit from, and it encourages an attitude of abundance over scarcity. No rigidity is required.

Flexibility

Life doesn't always go to plan, and sometimes (or often) it calls for us to go with the flow. Let's say you plan to make a home-cooked meal after work, but you have a stressful day, and it's the last thing you want to do when you get home. In this case, would it be more or less stressful for you to follow through with your original plan? Gentle nutrition calls for us to be flexible and understand that perfection does not exist, nor is it required to be healthy — remember the 'zooming out' strategy I mentioned previously. We need to take eating into the context of our overall diet and lifestyle. Sometimes it's more important to throw on a frozen pizza or ready meal if it serves you better. Your eating will naturally shift in response to what life throws at you, and that's OK. Flexibility over rigidity always. Learning to embrace flexibility and imperfection is a key part of integrating nutrition without a side of diet culture.

Self-care

Sometimes you need to do the best you can with the resources you have, which may mean that food is used as self-care. For example, while I am finishing the book you are holding in your hands, I may not be able to spend as much time as I usually would on meal prep. Self-care for me during that time will be allowing myself to order a takeaway instead of putting myself under pressure to spend time cooking a meal. Likewise, it may also mean that food is used as one tool in your coping-skills toolkit, and that's also OK. We all emotionally eat from time to time, and as long as we stay present and pay attention to what's going on, this isn't a case for alarm.

The Five Fundamentals

I have a super-easy formula to help with building out nutritionally balanced meals. I use this system, albeit subconsciously at this stage, every time I go to make a meal or walk into a supermarket. Keeping the five fundamentals in mind is a sure-fire way to create nutritionally balanced meals every time. You should aim to include each of the five fundamentals in every meal. Remember to approach this with flexibility over rigidity — not all meals will contain all five and that's OK as long as they are in the majority of your meals. I like to use the 'zooming out' technique when incorporating nutrition guidelines. No one food or meal will make or break your health. It's important to look at your diet as a whole rather than individually assessing each meal or snack.

1. Carbohydrates
Carbohydrates are the body's preferred source of fuel and provide us with energy. If you cut carbohydrates out of your diet, you will feel hungry. Very hungry. Remember NPY, the 'carb fairy' hormone I referred to in Chapter 6? Every meal should contain carbohydrates to ensure your energy needs are being met — there is no equal substitute for carbohydrates. The below table contains a list of some starchy and non-starchy carbohydrates. Starchy carbs provide energy so these must

284

be included in every meal – non-starchy carbohydrates alone are not enough. Carbohydrates are also an important source of fibre, an essential compound for health and vitality, which I will cover more when we discuss blood sugar balance.

Starchy carbohydrates	Non-starchy carbohydrates
Bread	Broccoli
Potatoes	Leafy greens
Pasta	Peppers
Rice	Spinach
Couscous	Mushrooms
Bulgar wheat	Celery
Barley	Tomato
Oats	Carrots

2. Protein

Protein provides the body with the building blocks it requires and is mainly responsible for growth and repair. We need amino acids, the small molecules that proteins are composed of, for everything from facilitating chemical reactions in the body to building muscles and organs to forming the structure of our DNA. Unlike carbohydrates and fats, protein hasn't been demonized by diet culture and has instead been put on a pedestal. Yes, protein is very important, but we don't need as much protein as you may think. It's currently estimated that the average adult requires about 0.8 kilos of protein per kilo of body weight each day. Luckily, in the Western world, people tend to meet their protein requirements easily, especially if a source of protein is included in each meal. Protein can be found in both animal and plant sources, as shown in the examples below.

Animal sources	Plant sources
Meat	Beans
Fish	Lentils
Turkey	Nuts
Chicken	Seeds
Milk	Peas
Eggs	Tofu
Cheese	Meat alternatives
Other dairy products	Soy

3. Fat

Fat is an essential macronutrient and dietary fat plays an important role in the body. It helps us to absorb fat-soluble vitamins (A, D, E, and K), keeps us warm and helps to protect our internal organs. Not only that, but fat carries flavour, which means that it also plays an important role in satisfaction – fat is what makes food taste good. Diet culture has demonized fat, just like it has demonized carbohydrates, but fat should not be feared. There are two main types of fat in the food we eat: saturated and unsaturated, the sources of which are listed in the table on the next page. If you consume a diet high in saturated fat, it can increase your risk of heart disease and stroke, but this does not mean it needs to be cut out completely. You can be mindful of your consumption, especially if you have a family history of hypertension, high cholesterol, heart disease, or stroke, without being too rigid and controlled about it.

Unsaturated fats can be further broken down into mono-unsaturated and polyunsaturated fats. Polyunsaturated fats help to lower LDL cholesterol (the type that increases heart-disease risk) and can be further broken down into the essential fatty acids omega-3 and -6, which need to be consumed from the diet. We tend to get plenty of omega-6 in the Western diet but much less omega-3, meaning that, generally, most people need to try and consume more of this. Omega-3 can be found in oily fish such as salmon, mackerel, and herring, and in plant-based sources such as flaxseeds and walnuts, although the plant-based sources are less bioavailable than the animal sources. Bioavailability refers to the ability of a substance to be absorbed and used by the body. A higher proportion of unsaturated fats to saturated fats is recommended for health and vitality.

When it comes to adding fats to mealtimes as part of the five fundamentals formula, they may not be always visible on the plate. For example, they could be in the butter you mash into your potatoes, the olive oil you roast your vegetables in, or the omega-3 in a piece of salmon.

Saturated fats	Unsaturated fats
Meat	Oily fish (salmon, mackerel, herring)
Processed meats	Avocado
Dairy	Nuts
Egg yolks	Seeds
Coconut oil	Olive oil
Cakes	Olives
Desserts	Rapeseed oil

4. *Fruits and/or vegetables*

If there's one piece of advice that tends to be universally accepted, it's that we all need to increase our consumption of fruit and vegetables. Overall, eating more plants in general is a good guideline to live by, since they are such an important source of fibre, micronutrients, and antioxidants. Antioxidants are chemicals that lessen or prevent the effects of free radicals – waste substances produced by cells as the body processes food and reacts to the environment. These free radicals can cause oxidative stress, leading to cell damage and death. Oxidative stress, an excess of free radicals in the body, causes inflammation in the body and in turn, may play a role in the development of a range of different health conditions, including cancer.[3] Antioxidants act like 'free radical scavengers' that mop up any damage. Free radical production is an inescapable part of life, but we can lessen its impact by eating more plants. Every meal should contain a fruit or vegetable — not just as a dressing, but as a substantial part of the meal. Eating more plants will only benefit you because of the incredible power they hold (I'm such a nerdy nutritionist with how excited I get about fruits and vegetables!)

Contrary to popular belief, five portions of fruit and vegetables a day is the minimum we should aim for, not the upper limit, with some studies suggesting that ten a day is the optimum quantity! If you can have more than five a day, great. Just do your best, knowing that more is often better (within reason). The list below is far from exhaustive but contains some examples of fruit and vegetables to begin including in your meals.

Fruits	Vegetables
Apples	Carrots
Pears	Parsnips
Oranges	Peppers
Berries	Broccoli
Melon	Beetroot
Kiwis	Courgette
Grapes	Cucumber
Banana	Aubergine
Mango	Lettuce
Avocado	Onion

5. Flavour
Last, but definitely not least, is flavour. When I began my career, I spent many years working alongside chefs, helping to improve the nutritional quality of the food on offer in their restaurants. As you can imagine, flavour is top of the priority list for chefs – as it should be! Flavour is key to satisfaction, and as you now know, satisfaction is an important part of a healthy relationship with food. It's possible for a meal to contain both flavour and health benefits – the two are not mutually exclusive. I feel as though diet culture has left a sour taste in the mouths of many by removing flavour from food, all in the name of 'health'. This has left many people with the belief that healthy food does not equal tasty food, which couldn't be further from the truth. If food tastes good, we are more likely to feel satisfied and choose that food again and again. If it doesn't taste good, we are unlikely to do so long term. It's really that simple.

The Five Fundamentals in Action

Here's an example of a straightforward meal to demonstrate the five fundamentals at work:

- ☐ Carbohydrate – potatoes
- ☐ Protein – roast chicken
- ☐ Fat – drizzle of olive oil
- ☐ Vegetables – carrots and broccoli
- ☐ Flavour – gravy

This meal contains each of the five fundamentals, meaning that it is nutritionally balanced. If you ensure your meals include a carbohydrate, protein, and fat source, alongside a fruit or vegetable and some flavour to boot, you'll be well on your way toward hitting your nutritional needs.

Blood Sugar Balance

Maintaining blood sugar balance throughout the day is vital for stable energy levels. Imbalanced blood sugar levels can profoundly impact your energy, mood, and ability to meet the demands of daily life and, if chronically mismanaged, can wreak havoc on your long-term health. The primary macro-nutrient that affects your blood sugar levels and, therefore, your energy levels are carbohydrates, which makes sense, given that it is recommended that 45 to 60 per cent of energy comes from carbohydrates. When you eat a food containing carbo-hydrates, during digestion it is broken down into glucose molecules, the compound that causes an increase in blood sugar levels. When this happens, the hypothalamus detects this rise, reduces the release of the hunger hormone ghrelin, and stimulates the release of the fullness hormone leptin, signalling to the body that you can stop eating. When your blood sugar levels dip below a level the body feels comfortable at, and there is no longer enough short-term glucose circulating in the bloodstream, you will begin to feel hungry, dizzy, shaky, and fatigued. You may start obsessing about food or dreaming about cookies, chocolate, or soft drinks — for a very under-standable reason. These foods contain simple carbohydrates and release their energy quickly, meaning that the glucose the body is craving will hit the bloodstream all at once. So there is a physiological reason you crave foods like chocolate, bread and pasta when your energy levels dip – it's not a character flaw. This is why if you are trying to improve your habits around food, it's essential to work on balancing your blood sugar levels.

Balancing your meals using the five fundamentals formula and eating regularly will help keep your blood sugar levels stable, but the quality of the carbohydrates you consume can also help with this. As well as being starchy or non-starchy, carbohydrates are often referred to as simple carbohydrates and complex carbohydrates. Simple carbohydrates release their energy quickly. Complex carbohydrates release their energy slowly. This is one of the reasons why wholegrain carbo-hydrates, such as brown bread, pasta, and rice, are recommended as part of healthy eating guidelines. Since wholegrain carbs contain more fibre than their white counter-parts, they take longer to be digested, and their energy hits the bloodstream more steadily. This does not mean that white versions of carbohydrates are 'bad' or that they need to be cut out, but being conscious of this and choosing wholegrain where possible will support stable blood sugar levels and, therefore, how you feel in your mind and body.

How Does Food Make You Feel?

To uncover your unique nutritional needs, pay attention to how food makes you feel. Rather than relying on external judgements of whether a food is considered 'good' or 'bad', check in with how different foods feel in your body. Pay atten-tion to how they affect your energy levels, concentration, digestion, and mood. Doing this will allow you to regain control over your eating decisions because the answer to whether a food is 'good' or 'bad' for you lies within. For example, I love the taste of pizza, but I don't always enjoy how I feel in my body afterwards. This doesn't mean that I never eat pizza, but it does inform my decision of whether or not to choose it. Sometimes I will, sometimes I won't, depending on how I feel in my body and how I wish to feel after a meal. Once you have rebuilt trust with your body by following the guidelines outlined in the previous chapters, checking in with how food makes you feel will become much easier. To help you uncover this, you can ask yourself the below questions:

How does this food make my body feel while I'm eating it?

Do I like this feeling?

How do I feel after I eat it?

Would I choose to feel this way again?

To take this further, you can use the rating systems below to monitor how you feel after eating certain foods.

On a scale of 1–10, did this meal or food make me feel:

Lethargic 1 – – – – – – – – – 10 Energetic

Heavy 1 – – – – – – – – – 10 Light

Dissatisfied 1 – – – – – – – – – 10 Satisfied

Distracted 1 – – – – – – – – – 10 Focused

Unwell 1 – – – – – – – – – 10 Well

By using the mindfulness skills you have learnt about in this book, you will begin to build up a bank of food experiences to guide your future food choices. Ultimately, the end goal is to nourish your body and feel amazing as a result — all while allowing all foods in without restriction and experiencing true food freedom. Who wouldn't want that?

Making Space for More Than One Truth

When people have moved through phases one (remove) and two (reconnect) of healing their relationship with food, and they come to the point of integrating nutrition knowledge into their food choices, confusion can arise. People often ask me, 'How can I start looking at nutrition without a side of diet culture?' I get it. You might once again be engaging in some behaviours that were present in your dieting days, which may feel scary. But the difference here is your mindset and intention. You no longer have the all-or-nothing mindset of diet culture. You are not engaging in these behaviours purely just for weight loss. Suppose you feel stuck with this and cannot seem to begin embracing health-promoting behaviours without once again falling into dietland. In that case, I recommend reaching out to a non-diet nutritionist or dietician for support.

So how do we begin to integrate nutrition and health values with an intuitive eating mindset? Regarding food, nutrition, and health, we need to embrace the fact that we can simultaneously hold two truths about something. For example:

☐ Sweets can be included in a healthy diet AND eating too many of them can cause tooth decay.

- ☐ We can enjoy foods high in saturated fat without guilt AND be conscious that consuming a high quantity of these is likely to increase the risk of heart disease.

- ☐ White carbohydrates are delicious AND they tend to be lower in fibre than wholemeal carbohydrates.

- ☐ Fizzy drinks may be enjoyed as part of a healthy diet AND they have a high glycaemic index, which can cause blood sugar peaks and troughs.

- ☐ We can allow all foods in without restriction AND choose some foods over others because of their impact on our health.

- ☐ Weight is largely genetically determined AND we can influence it to an extent through the diet and lifestyle we choose to engage in.

A certain amount of letting go and taking responsibility is required in making changes to truly benefit your health, physically, mentally, emotionally and spiritually. On the one hand, you need to let go of the need to control things you cannot control, but on the other hand, you need to take responsibility for the things that you can change, the things that you can control, that will influence both your weight and your health. But you need to have the ability to take responsibility, and this may not always be possible during challenging times, such as periods of stress or overwhelm. It's not always straightforward. If this is the case and you're feeling very stuck, I recommend reaching out for professional support.

Affirmations

I nourish my body with nutritious food.

I prioritize feeling good in my body.

I use brain and body knowledge to make food choices.

I release dietary perfection and embrace flexibility.

I consider how food will make me feel.

I make nutritional additions to my meals and snacks.

Chapter 14:

Movement

'Come to yoga, I think it'll be really good for you.'

It was 2017. My good friend Jenna knew I was going through a hard time and she convinced me to join her at a weekly yoga class she attended. (I really do have the best friends.) My relationship with exercise up to this point was rocky, to say the least. I hated it with a passion. I was like a perpetual dieter when it came to exercise. For years, ever since the age of sixteen, I had used exercise for one thing and one thing only — to change my body. I had tried everything: running, swimming, gymming, bums-and-tums classes, boot camp — you name it, I'd tried it. But yoga? Never. I was a bit cynical, if I'm being honest, and worried that I wouldn't fit in. Back then, I thought yoga sounded 'a bit strange' and was just for those 'weird hippies'. How ironic that I now consider myself one of those people — don't knock it till you try it!

With all the different forms of exercise I had tried over the years, nothing ever stuck. I felt like a complete failure and had just resigned myself to the fact that exercise wasn't for me and that was never going to change. So many times I'd tried something new, and been super excited and motivated about it, until a week later I began to dread it, and it all fell apart once again. Until next time. I believed that it would always be something I had to make myself do, a chore. I know this will resonate with some of you.

I think my fractured relationship with exercise started quite young, when I was in primary school and was forced to engage in exercise I disliked. This is nobody's fault — schools do the best they can with the resources they have. Nonetheless, the negative experience I had stayed with me and shaped my relationship with exercise as I got older. I am not a sporty person — I never played football or camogie or any of the other sports some of my friends played in school. PE, or physical education, is taught to all Irish children from primary school age — usually from age five. For me, this meant learning how to play football — my worst nightmare in school. I can still remember those days out on the football pitch, in the wind and the rain, with little balls of cotton wool stuffed into my ears underneath a woolly hat. I had very sensitive ears as a child and experienced intense inner ear pain when exposed to the wind (which is still the case today). Naturally, I began to despise PE — i.e. exercise — and everything associated with it. This negative association that formed in early childhood led to the development of a core belief: 'I hate exercise.' This core belief was only strengthened as I moved into my teenage years, as every form of exercise I tried and disliked gave me more evidence to support it. There are reasons for this, which I will be discussing later on in this chapter.

So, why I am sharing this insight into my personal relationship with exercise? Well, because firstly, just as your relationship with food develops over time and is influenced by your environment, your upbringing, your weight, and your past experiences, so too is your relationship with exercise. If you find it hard to engage with exercise, it's important to look back at your history to examine what has shaped your perception of it. Only then can you truly understand what went wrong and therefore, what you can begin to change going forward.

The change for me happened in that first-ever yoga class I attended. I remember walking in filled with the fear and anticipation that comes from entering a room full of strangers, not knowing what to expect. I found myself a mat in the back corner and hoped it wouldn't be yet another form of exercise to dislike. My experience was anything but, and I was hooked from that first class. I felt physically challenged, but mentally calm – I had never experienced anything like it. That first yoga class liberated me from the thoughts and feelings I had about exercise. It rattled my core belief of 'I hate exercise.' It changed everything. I grew to love movement when previously it had been a chore. Yoga is now my peace that can weather any storm and has become a constant in my life, always there to support me. It helped me connect with my mind, body, and inner self in a way that no other form of movement allowed. This element of connection now greatly informs my career as a nutritionist and, within that, in helping people to become healthier, happier versions of themselves. My yoga training and personal practice have played and continue to play a huge role in how I work with my clients on a daily basis. After that first class, I attended religiously every week (travelling from Dublin to Carlow every Thursday to do so), before going on to my 200-hour training and then two 30-hour trainings to specialize in and learn about the magic of yin yoga. If you had told me back in 2016 that I would one day become a yoga teacher, I would have laughed in your face. My relationship with exercise completely transformed, and if I can do it, so can you.

Movement over Exercise

When I speak about exercise throughout the rest of this chapter, I will be referring to it as movement, or I may use the words exercise and movement interchangeably. There is nothing wrong with the word 'exercise', and I have no problem describing movement in this way, but unfortunately, for a lot of us, the word 'exercise' comes with many negative associations, such as the personal ones I described at the start of this chapter. I see both ends of the spectrum in clinic: either people have a complete aversion to exercise or they are over-exercising. For many of my clients, exercise is synonymous with a chore, something that has to be done, no matter what. From my experience, it's associated with pain or struggle and is less likely to be associated with joy and pleasure. It's often heavily associated with weight loss or is used solely as a means to reshape the body. Also, movement is generally only considered exercise in the minds of many if it's of a certain intensity. For example, a stroll to enjoy nature is not typically considered exercise, but a power walk is.

When a new client comes to work with me, I always ask them about their relationship with exercise. One past client, let's call her Jane, told me that she never exercised consistently and she felt very ashamed about it. She shared that she just couldn't seem to stick to anything, even though she knew how great exercise made her feel. Her story was very similar to mine. Once we began to dig a little bit deeper, I discovered that she cycled to work every day — fifteen minutes each way. That's thirty minutes of exercise she was getting, five days a week, which the WHO recommends as the minimum level of weekly physical activity. When I shared this with her, she couldn't comprehend it, as she said that cycling was just part of her day. She had never considered it as exercise. But it doesn't have to kill you to count.

Movement, as a word, is broader than exercise. It's more inclusive. Since it's a new word to describe exercise for many, there are fewer negative associations attached to it. Language is very powerful, and in this case it can be harnessed for good. Here are some examples of what movement could look like:

- ☐ A stroll on the beach

- ☐ A power walk

- ☐ A slow and gentle yoga class

- ☐ A strong and dynamic yoga class

- ☐ A run

- ☐ A jog

- ☐ Running around after the kids or grandkids

- ☐ Walking to the local shop

- [ ] Going for a hike

- [ ] Hoovering the house

- [ ] Gardening

- [ ] Playing with the dog

- [ ] Cycling to work

As this list demonstrates, when it comes to movement everything counts. It doesn't have to feel like torture to be worthwhile.

What Is Intuitive Movement?

Intuitive movement is all about flexibility rather than rigidity around exercise. It's about letting go of rules and regulations, shoulds and have-tos. It is an approach to movement that places joy as the dominant motivator. It allows you to listen to your own body and the messages from within to guide you to the type, quantity, and intensity of exercise that feels good for you on any given day. In the words of Tally Rye, an intuitive movement fitness coach, intuitive movement is 'the practice of building trust with your body so you can make the right decisions as to which type of movement is best for you – along with the right decisions about intensity, duration and rest'.

We all have different physical abilities, fitness levels, likes and dislikes, time demands, responsibilities, goals and values. Intuitive movement makes space for these differences, as your relationship with movement is as unique as your relationship with food. With intuitive movement, there is no such thing as one form of exercise being better than another — everything is worthwhile. Diet culture infiltrates how we see exercise and tells us things like:

'If you don't sweat, it doesn't count.'

'You have to push yourself to your absolute limit.'

'No pain, no gain.'

'The harder, the better.'

I don't know about you, but none of these things ever landed very well with me or encouraged my relationship with movement — they made me hate exercise and see it as torture. I remember being forced to do a certain number of push-ups in an exercise class, or else the whole room would be punished. It was my first time at this class and my physical ability was less than many others in the room. Needless to say, I never went back! I'm all for pushing yourself at times — I often have to push myself to go to a yoga class on days that I'm feeling lazy, but other times my body really is tired and I need a rest. Intuitive movement allows me to honour those needs. You are the only person who knows your edge. Playing that edge is key to developing more strength and stamina, but if you push yourself beyond your limit, there's a good chance you will injure yourself or grow tired of exercise altogether.

Why Exercise Becomes a Chore . . .

There are many reasons why exercise may have become a chore for you and, as a result, something you don't want to do. Here are some of the reasons I have seen, both through my own experience and that of my clients.

All-or-nothing mindset

When we approach something with an all-or-nothing mindset, it leaves very little room for the eventualities of life. An all-or-nothing mindset might work out if we were robots, living in little bubbles that weren't affected by anything outside of us, but that's not the case. Since life doesn't always go according to plan, so too should you extend that possibility to your plans around movement. By approaching your movement routine with flexibility, instead of rigidity, it is more likely to become a sustainable habit.

Setting unrealistic goals

Setting unrealistic goals is a hallmark of approaching exercise with a diet mentality. It usually has a flavour of 'I'm going to go to the gym five days a week for an hour each time.' This may be a realistic goal for some, and that's great, but often when you're starting something new, it's not a good idea to go straight from zero to a hundred. Instead, it's better to build up your movement habit over time. Pair an unrealistic goal with an all-or-nothing mindset, and you've got a recipe for failure. If your goal sounds even a small bit unrealistic, it's a sign you need to re-evaluate.

Lack of enjoyment

Think of something you hate doing. Now think about having to do that five times a week for the rest of your life. How does that feel? What kind of response does it elicit? I'll bet it's not a positive one. Movement is no different. If you dislike the form of movement you are trying to engage with, it won't last long. Enjoyment and pleasure are absolutely essential for long-term sustainability.

Lack of intrinsic motivation
Intrinsic motivation is key for maintaining a health-promoting behaviour. Unlike extrinsic motivation, where the main motivators are external rewards, intrinsic motivation refers to behaviour that is driven by internal rewards. You engage with the behaviour purely for internal satisfaction. The behaviour itself is the reward. When related to movement, these internal rewards can be found in how you feel during and after exercise, or how it affects your mood, sleep, or general temperament. Would you exercise even if it meant your body never changed? If your answer is no, this is a sign of a hyper focus on extrinsic motivation and a lack of intrinsic motivation. Extrinsic motivation alone will not maintain a consistent movement routine.

Linked to weight loss or body reshaping
Using exercise purely as a means to lose weight or shape your body in a particular way is a form of extrinsic motivation. When movement is linked to weight loss, you are not engaging in the behaviour because you enjoy it and find it satisfying, but because you expect something in return: weight loss. When weight loss is the main motivator, it also increases the likelihood that the reasons discussed above will creep into your relationship with movement, as you push harder to succeed and earn the reward of losing

weight for your efforts. And if that doesn't happen or to the extent you hope . . . well, you know what happens then. The movement stops.

. . . And What to Do About It

Do any of the above points resonate with you, or can you spot them in your own relationship with movement? Luckily, there are steps you can take to rebuild your relationship with exercise and embrace intuitive movement. Intuitive movement allows your body to be your guide. Instead of relying upon external opinions about what the 'best' way is to exercise, you check in with yourself to answer that question. By checking in with how you feel, physically, mentally, and emotionally, you will be guided to the answers of what kind of movement would feel best in your body. This can change from day to day, week to week, month to month, and season to season. We are not robots and our energy levels fluctuate, which significantly impacts the kind of movement (or rest) required to satisfy those needs.

Find something you enjoy
Let's start with the basics. You need to find some form of movement that you genuinely enjoy. If you hate to run, fine, don't choose running as your movement of choice. Don't be afraid to get out there and try new things without attaching to any particular outcome. You might like it, or you might not. The outcome doesn't matter. You will only find something you do enjoy by exploring the different movement options available to you.

Set realistic goals
Setting unrealistic goals is a hallmark sign of diet mentality. Start small and build up your goals over time. Setting small, manageable goals you know you can hit helps build the momentum and confidence you need to set more ambitious ones. It doesn't matter how small your realistic goals sound to you — they may even pale in comparison to the goals you set for yourself in the past. See this as a good sign that you are listening to what is actually attainable and taking steps to move away from the diet mentality dictating your relationship with movement.

Release any and all expectations
When it comes to setting goals for movement, I have what I like to call a 'get out of jail free card'. Let's say you choose walking as your movement of choice, and your goal is to walk three times a week. Laying expectations onto this goal could look like:

☐ Walking for one hour

☐ Working up a sweat

☐ Walking five kilometres

There's absolutely nothing wrong with setting any of the above as goals; however, being rigid and inflexible with them doesn't allow for changes in your energy levels or the impact of other factors that may prevent you from reaching them. What if you're too tired to walk for an hour? Or your ankle starts to hurt when you're halfway through your five-kilometre walk? Or if you get sick? There has to be room for you to listen to the needs of the body, which is why dropping any and all expectations and just going with the flow is key. This can make the difference between grabbing your runners and getting out the door vs collapsing on the couch to watch Netflix. Setting a goal when you wake up to walk for an hour that evening might seem manageable after a great night's sleep, but it may seem impossible when the time comes and you've just got home from a challenging day at work. But fifteen minutes may seem more accessible. Without having flexibility and releasing expectations of yourself, it's unlikely that fifteen minutes will be 'good enough'.

For example, I set myself a goal to practise yoga multiple times a week, but I check in with my body on a daily basis and ask myself, 'Do I need something gentle and relaxing today or do I need something fast and invigorating?' At the start of the week, I have no idea what I'll need tomorrow or the next day. When I get on my mat, I have no idea how long I'll be there (with the exception of when I attend a class), because I am listening to my body from moment to moment. Sometimes it will be fifteen minutes, sometimes it will be an hour. Everything is worthwhile. Everything counts.

Set yourself up for success
Setting yourself up for success means putting things in place that make it as easy as possible to make movement a part of your day. This could look like:

☐ Laying out your gym clothes the night before

☐ Putting your yoga mat in the car

☐ Having extra fitness equipment in the house

☐ Ensuring you have comfortable clothes and foot-wear to exercise in

☐ Blocking out time in your calendar for movement

☐ Planning adequate childcare if needed

☐ Making exercise plans with friends

Ask yourself, 'What would this look like if it were easy?'

Be compassionate with yourself
Shame does not make you do better. Berating yourself does not work. Be kind to yourself, especially if you are reintegrating movement into your life. Your fitness level may not be where you'd like it or where it was in the past, and that's OK. You will improve and get better, but you cannot do that if you do not give yourself compassion and allow yourself to fail, especially if you are trying something new. Putting yourself out there and trying to improve is a massive win — give yourself credit and compassion.

Listen to your body
Last, but definitely not least, allow yourself to listen to the messages of your body. Let your body be your guide. If your body needs rest, allow yourself to rest. If you're feeling sluggish, stiff, and fatigued, more movement may be just the ticket. If you find yourself in an exercise class, out for a walk, or on a run and you've hit your limit or lost your breath, allow yourself to take a break. Your body is giving you a constant

flow of messages when you move. Listening to them will allow you to provide the body what it needs, moment to moment.

Finding Your Joy

If you dread exercise, it's a sign that you may not be engaging in joyful movement. Is there any form of movement that you genuinely enjoy? That is, one that you don't tell yourself you enjoy but secretly hate? If the answer is no, then we've got some exploration to do. How exciting! And that's precisely what finding a form of movement you enjoy can feel like.

Before you think that's impossible, remember this is coming from a self-confessed past hater of exercise. When you embark on an intuitive movement journey, especially if you are coming to it with the experience of intense and unsustainable exercise regimes, it can be challenging to know where to start. Allow yourself to play and have fun again by moving your body. Have you ever watched kids outside playing? They have bucketloads of energy and will run around all day. Technically, this is exercise, but we only begin to call it that when we move into adulthood. Why? Why does exercise become something we 'must' and 'should' do when we grow up? Why can't it continue to be something we do for fun?

I remember having a conversation with a past client about intuitive movement and explaining that there are lots of different forms of movement she could begin to try out. She told me that she had been mountain biking with her brother the weekend before, but because it was for fun, she never considered it exercise! If it's fun and involves you moving your body, you've hit the absolute jackpot!

If you're feeling lost, ask yourself what kind of movement sounds like something you would enjoy if exercise didn't affect what your body looked like on the outside. Try some different movement classes, such as yoga, Pilates, barre, aerobics, dance, spin, kick-boxing and so on, or get outside and try hiking, walking, tennis, squash, paddle, surfing, or snow-boarding. Don't forget to switch it up to have a bit of variety. Remember that everyday activities like playing with the dog, running around after the kids, hoovering, cleaning the house, gardening, or walking to work also count.

Now, go out there and find your joy with movement – that's your only requirement!

The Benefits of Movement

The benefits of adding more movement to your life are endless. For starters, a regular exercise routine can lead to several different health-risk reductions:

☐ Cognitive decline

☐ Colon cancer

☐ Depression

☐ Endometrial cancer

☐ Heart disease

☐ Hypertension

☐ Insulin resistance

☐ Lung cancer

- ☐ Osteoporosis and bone fractures
- ☐ Premature death
- ☐ Stroke
- ☐ Type 2 diabetes

It can also lead to many long-term health outcomes, such as improved:

- ☐ Bone density
- ☐ Grey matter of brain
- ☐ Cognition and memory
- ☐ Gut microbiota
- ☐ Satiety cues
- ☐ Lean body mass
- ☐ Cardiovascular circulation

Along with short-term health benefits, such as improved:

- ☐ Strength
- ☐ Balance
- ☐ Mood
- ☐ Stamina
- ☐ Appetite regulation

☐ Stress tolerance

☐ Sleep quality

If you have ever engaged in consistent exercise, you will know the potential that movement has to make you feel amazing. In order to reap all of the benefits above, you need to move your body regularly and consistently. When exercise is tied to dieting or weight loss, it's likely to be less enjoyable and therefore you will be less motivated to engage with it consistently. This is why it's so important to detach movement from weight loss and instead focus on how it makes you feel.

So how much movement do you need to do? The World Health Organization recommends:

150 minutes/2 hours 30 minutes
per week of moderate activity
(for example, walking, gardening)

or

75 minutes of vigorous activity
(for example, hiking, tennis, jogging)

+

Two muscle-strengthening activities
(for example, yoga, weight-lifting)

This is not to say that you can't do more — it is the minimum requirement for health. This is not a rule but a guideline you can take into consideration when planning to engage in a more regular exercise routine. Doing some physical activity is better than none, so start small and just get moving in whatever way you find joyful.

Let Your Body Be Your Guide

Rather than relying on calorie or fitness trackers to define the value of movement, let your body be your guide. How does movement make you feel? The key to a consistent exercise routine is to tune into how exercise feels in your body both during and after. For example, I practise yoga because it makes my body feel strong, my mind feel calm, and I sleep like a baby afterwards – especially if I've attended a hot class! This is why I practise yoga consistently and continue to return to my mat – these reasons are intrinsic and not extrinsic. After you exercise, check in with the below:

Stress: do you handle stress better? Are you less on edge?

Energy: do you feel more alert or energetic?

Sleep: do you sleep better?

Mood: does your mind feel clearer? Do you feel happier or more optimistic?

Body: does your body feel stronger? Does it feel more mobile or lighter? Do you have a pep in your step?

You should also check in with your energy levels from day to day to allow your body to guide you to the form of movement (or rest) you require. To do this, ask yourself:

What does my body need today?

What type of movement do I feel like doing today?

What type of exercise would best support what my body needs today?

Some days, I will need an intense vinyasa flow yoga class to feel energized and strong. On other days, I will need a relaxing yin class or a short walk in nature. Our energy levels are not the same every day, so we shouldn't expect our exercise routine to be the same. Allow yourself to listen to your body to guide you to what you need most.

The Power of Yoga

Yoga has changed my life.

I used to roll my eyes when I heard people say things like this and think to myself, 'What does that even mean, and how the hell can something like yoga change your life?!' Then I experienced it for myself. Yoga is my calm that can weather any storm. It helps me to reconnect with my body in a way nothing else ever has. It helps me to access what is going on within, and I am often surprised at what I find when I practise. It has helped me to make huge decisions in my life and gain clarity on the next right step for me at many different crossroads. I have cried during yoga. I have laughed and felt anger, frustration, and disappointment. Yoga has taught me the skill of sitting with discomfort, something I have brought off the mat and into my everyday life. Of course, this can only truly be understood when it is experienced, but I am telling you this because of how powerful the practice is and how aligned it is with food and body image healing. I often say that yoga is to exercise like intuitive eating is to nutrition. Being a yoga teacher, I am, of course, biased, but for good reason. The practice of yoga encourages you to connect with the body and to move in an embodied way, something that by now you will understand is a core piece of rebuilding your relationship with food.

I am not suggesting that yoga is for everyone (although I do believe everyone could benefit from some form of it). Perhaps you dislike yoga but love running; that's OK. You need to find what works for you and we are all different, but I couldn't possibly write a book without speaking about yoga when I know how much potential it has to enhance a food and body image healing journey.

Yoga comes in many different forms — it can be as hard or as easy as you'd like it to be. Everybody can practise yoga. No matter your size, there is a place for you in yoga within the right environment and with the right teacher. Every teacher brings their own unique style when teaching a class, so you may need to shop around to find the style that you enjoy. To get you started, here are brief descriptions of some of the most popular forms of yoga:

☐ Hatha yoga — Postures held for time. Good for beginners.

☐ Vinyasa yoga — A fast-paced yoga class where you flow through postures in one-breath movements. Prepare to sweat.

☐ Yin-yang yoga — A blend of 'active' (yang) postures and 'passive' (yin) postures.

☐ Restorative yoga — Total chill, there will be no sweating in this class. Excellent for nervous-system regulation.

☐ Yin yoga — Relaxation with a challenge. No sweating, but prepare for deep stretches held for time. Also excellent for nervous-system regulation.

Yoga is so much more than a physical practice; for some, it is a deeply spiritual practice. There are eight limbs of yoga, and the physical movement of a yoga class makes up just one of these eight limbs.

1. Yama
This refers to moral disciplines or practices that are primarily concerned with the world around us and how we interact with It. There are five yamas: non-violence (ahimsa), truthfulness (satya), non-stealing (asteya), non-overindulgence (brahmacharya), and non-greed (aparigraha).

2. Niyama
The niyamas are personal observances concerned with the self and can be thought of as recommended habits for healthy living and spirituality. These include cleanliness (saucha), contentment (santosha), self-discipline (tapas), self-study (svadhyaya) and surrender to a higher power (ishvara pranidhana).

3. Asana

Asana, meaning 'posture' or 'seat', is the physical aspect of yoga and the one that most people are familiar with. Particularly in the West, asana practice (the physical postures of a yoga class) is needed to remove physical tensions, improve strength, and bring a busy mind to quietness.

4. Pranayama

This is the art and science of breathing, commonly described as breathwork. The breath is powerful and when harnessed can impact the mind and body in a beneficial way. Pranayama translates to 'breath-control', and the ability to slow down or retain the breath in or out of the body takes time and practice. Correct breathing is of immense importance and essential to asana practice.

5. Pratyahara

Pratyahara refers to the withdrawal of the senses. In practice, this means to draw your attention inwards, which may include focusing on the breath. Instead of actually losing the ability to hear, smell, see, touch, and taste, we become so absorbed in what it is we are focusing on that we become less easily distracted.

6. Dharana

Dharana means 'focused concentration'. The deeper our concentration, the clearer and more at peace the mind will become. This is closely linked to pratyahara, since to concentrate on something, we must withdraw the senses. Visualization and pranayama exercises require the application of dharana.

7. *Dhyana*

The seventh limb refers to meditation — specifically, meditative absorption. This is when we become completely absorbed in the meditation itself. It brings about awareness without focus and moves us from a state of doing to being.

8. *Samadhi*

Samadhi, the final limb of yoga, means 'bliss' or 'enlightenment'. Once we have reorganized our relationship with both the inner and outer world, we come to the finale of bliss.

*

Yoga can be seen as a lifestyle, rather than simply physical movement. This is why it is often referred to as a practice. The eight limbs show us how we can bring the yoga that we practise in a class off the mat and into our lives. It encourages us to connect and reflect upon what is going on both inside and outside of ourselves. Personally, I see yoga as a spiritual practice, one that doesn't end and will most likely continue to deepen in nature as I move through life. For some, it is mainly a physical practice to improve strength, flexibility, and mobility, which is perfectly acceptable. This is the power of yoga — it has the potential to become what you make it. If it appeals to you, I highly recommend giving it a shot to deepen your journey of connection to the self.

Affirmations

I am becoming stronger every day.

Discomfort is a normal and expected part of change.

Any and all forms of movement count.

I offer myself compassion on my fitness journey.

I overcome fitness challenges with ease.

I let go of all expectation.

Real-Life Stories:

The Power of Lived Experience

In the following pages are some real-life stories from a few of my clients about their journey with intuitive eating and rebuilding their relationship with food. I just wish I could have included more! These real-life experiences are beautiful demonstrations of what is truly possible when you commit to rebuilding your relationship with food and body image. My goal in sharing these stories is to fill you with the hope that you, too, can achieve food freedom and to provide some words of wisdom from those who have walked the path before you. I have to thank my amazing clients who agreed to put their time and energy into writing these pieces so I could share them with you. You know who you are, and I am forever grateful to all of you. Without you, my work and this book would never have been possible. You all inspire me every day.

Carly

'Everything I've learned throughout this journey has changed me into a person I only ever dreamed I could be in another life.'

When we talk about intuitive eating, we talk a lot about freedom: freedom from dieting and freedom from pressure to conform to society's idea of 'health'. The concept of freedom from something that was my whole life's purpose never crossed my mind. I truly believed that to be thin was to be healthy – and no one could tell me otherwise (or so I thought). The relief that comes with moving away from dieting and into intuitive eating is felt by many. But as a fat person, that freedom is experienced on a deeper and far more intense level. Moving through the principles of intuitive eating during my sessions with Niamh, I came to learn that I spent fifteen years hating my body and blaming myself because of my weight rather than blaming the culture that decided the only way to be healthy, beautiful, and worthy is to be thin.

Diet culture has a way of getting under your skin, and it lived in me for years when my time, energy, and money were consumed by it. Being gently guided out of that place and releasing all the blame I was placing on myself was the best thing that's ever happened to me. Intuitive eating is rooted in building a healthy relationship with food and body image, but it's about so much more for me. Everything I've learned throughout this journey has changed me into a person I only ever dreamed I could be in another life. I have time and space to do the things that serve me. I have the capacity for emotional growth and learning. I live an embodied, authentic life and I finally feel at home in myself.

Repairing your relationship with food and body image is not easy work – how can it be when it involves peeling back layers of our ingrained belief systems around dieting? This stuff is hard, and sometimes working through it means uncovering things you never expected to find. To me, this is the beauty of food therapy. As I said, it's about so much more than the food. It takes a lot of learning, unlearning and exploration. I've cried a lot of tears, but I've laughed just as much. It takes a long time to accept that, unlike dieting, there is no passing or failing with intuitive eating, only learning and growing. This creates a safe and gentle environment, which is essential for this healing.

If you're thinking about starting your intuitive eating journey, be gentle with yourself. Going easy on yourself from the get-go and allowing self-compassion to fill that space in you will go a long way. Work with an intuitive eating counsellor if you can; support from a professional in this field is vital, in my opinion, and was paramount for my journey. Trust the process (because you probably won't in the beginning!). Most importantly, know that you are worthy of living a full life, one free from dieting, and you can have that life – right now.

Lucy

'I am so much happier now with all of the free brain space I have from not worrying about food and diets!'

My experience with the intuitive eating process has been completely life-changing. It has been a long and emotional journey to undo over fifteen years' worth of damage to my relationship with food and body image. Discovering intuitive eating has been an awakening. Before I found Niamh and intuitive eating, I thought that I would be on a diet for the rest of my life. I could not understand why I binged so much. I went through every diet imaginable — wasting a lot of money in the process! My weight cycled constantly, and my body image was at an all-time low. It was all-consuming.

I now have freedom from dieting and I don't think that much about food at all. I don't wake up every morning planning my meals and counting calories for the day, I don't feel guilty eating foods I enjoy, and I add nourishment to my meals and enjoy what I eat, eating for satisfaction as well as nutrition. I recognize my hunger and fullness cues. I am in tune with my body in a way I can't ever remember being before. If I do overeat, I have the tools and self-awareness to recognize why. I don't hate my body; I accept and respect it. I went through fertility treatment, pregnancy, and birth in a bigger body and had nothing but love for what my body went through, how strong it is, and an appreciation for what it can do. I fear that this would not have been the case if I hadn't found intuitive eating, and those processes would have been a completely different experience for me. This process triggered a lot more in my life than just eating intuitively. I now prioritize self-care, attend counselling, and have a completely different outlook on life. I don't have it all figured out, but I am so much happier now with all of the free brain space I have from not worrying about food and diets!

If anyone is teetering on the edge of (diet) rock bottom I would urge them to take the plunge into intuitive eating and put in the work. It's not easy, it can be a long and uncomfortable process, but the journey of self-awareness and discovery is worth the work. I now have a daughter whom I want to raise to trust her body, respect it, and have a better and more intuitive relationship with food than I never had throughout my teenage and adult life. I can't thank Niamh enough for her help during this life-changing process.

Leanne

'Intuitive eating has given me so much freedom in my mind, my body, and overall life.'

I would describe intuitive eating as a process of self-discovery and learning how to come back to your natural self. For me, a large part of the journey involved learning about my emotions, triggers, and how I coped with these. I learned how everything I have experienced and taken in over my entire life has shaped my relationship to myself, my body, and food. The intuitive eating process first started when I read *Just Eat It* by Laura Thomas. I related to so much of it, but I thought I could just go on one more diet and then I would start intuitive eating 'properly'. It ended up being nearly two years of dieting, losing, and gaining weight until I circled back to intuitive eating and said enough is enough.

Intuitive eating has given me so much freedom in my mind, my body, and overall life. The biggest change for me, I think, is putting my energy into much more meaningful things. Instead of constantly worrying about what I will look like, if I will lose 'X' amount of weight, tracking steps and calories, I now spend my energy building relationships with friends and family, doing things I actually enjoy and those that feel good, instead of doing things for the sole purpose of weight loss.

My key pieces of advice if you are getting ready to embark on this journey are to:

1. Spend some time figuring out what your core values are. Journal on it, write them down, and create a visualization board that you can use to remind yourself of what is important when things feel wobbly.

2. Try to surround yourself with a community that is on the intuitive eating journey with you and experiencing the same things – there are amazing social media pages, intuitive eating groups, workshops, and events that you can follow and join in on the conversation.

3. If you have a menstrual cycle, be mindful that our hormones impact our body image, confidence, mood, energy, and appetite. Learning how you experience your cycle and how you can adapt your life to go with your flow can help you sail smoothly through each month.

Caoimhe

'Intuitive eating has absolutely changed my life forever.'

The intuitive eating process has been a rollercoaster, to be honest! I started working with Niamh, still secretly hoping to lose weight, but I was sick and tired of extreme dieting and needed something more sustainable. I didn't really know what I was getting myself into. I quickly realized that intuitive eating is an anti-diet approach. I had been dieting (counting calories) for five years, so this was scary, unknown territory and I was feeling excited yet apprehensive.

I think the best way to describe the intuitive eating process is with the healing spiral. I embarked on a journey to heal my relationship with food and body image. Sometimes I felt healed and sometimes I felt as though I had taken two steps forward and one step back.

The most important things I learned through the intuitive eating process were:

1. To trust myself and my hunger/satiety signals.

2. Health comes in every size.

3. All bodies are beautiful.

4. It's possible to let all foods in and release guilt.

5. My worth has nothing to do with my body size or weight.

6. Healing isn't linear.

7. Body confidence is achievable, and it looks sexy on everyone.

8. Food isn't 'good' or 'bad' — food has no moral value.

Intuitive eating has absolutely changed my life forever. Working with Niamh not only healed my relationship with food and my body image — it gave me back my life, my headspace, and compassion for myself. Before this, my mind was consumed by food, weight, and appearance. Now I have time to think, I'm kinder to myself, and I LOVE myself! It helped open my eyes to the power of advertising, societal pressures, patriarchy, and misogyny — all alive and well today. My life is better and my mental health has improved due to being kinder to myself about my body. I am now much better at tuning into my hunger and satiety signals, and I know when my body needs nourishment. I feel more at one with and more present in my body, rather than desperately wanting it to be different. Even my relationship with exercise has changed — I now exercise to feel good and do what I enjoy, not in a strict or disciplined manner to lose weight.

The best advice I could give to people reading this is to be patient with yourself and expect the ups and downs to come. Some days I wanted to shout from the rooftops about intuitive eating; I was so happy with the process! On other days I genuinely wanted to scream, shout, and cry! It's a rollercoaster of a relationship, but I am so glad I found this way of living. Diversify your social media feed, too — it helps to appreciate all bodies in all shapes and sizes. Niamh's body image hierarchy taught me a lot. Body love feels like a hard thing to reach, so instead start with body respect, then move to body acceptance, and then to body love. Sometimes you will have bad body image days — even when you have reached body love! That's OK. That's normal!

Katie

'It's never too early or too late to start this journey — just start it.'

After I first heard about intuitive eating, I read the intuitive eating book and I listened to all the podcasts I could, but it took me a full year to commit to talking to a professional and prioritizing the cost of this. Talking to a professional was an essential part of the intuitive eating process for me and helped to consolidate what I had learned from books and podcasts and relate that information directly to my own life and experiences. Niamh helped me talk about all of the intricacies of my own life and apply the principles of intuitive eating in a way I hadn't been fully able to on my own. I went into the process thinking I needed only to work on my relationship with food and ended up realizing that there were so many areas of my life (relationships, self-care, boundaries, to name a few) that impacted my food decisions. I was surprised at how emotional I became in the accepting space created by Niamh and the vulnerability I felt in talking about food, which previously I had felt was quite a factual topic. It is one thing reading about self-compassion, but the one-to-one sessions with Niamh where I directly experienced that compassion and atmosphere of non-judgement were very powerful. It was freeing, and I felt a sense of relief after talking things through in every session. I have learned that I required the repetition of these sessions to fully change my habits and my thinking around food. I took so many insights and tips away from each meeting that I could practically implement in my daily life.

It is not an exaggeration to say that it has changed my life for the better. It has completely upended my relationship with food. I have such freedom and ease around food, both with myself and in situations where there are gatherings of people centred around food (for example, dinner with friends, parties). I can make decisions based on more important factors than 'weight' or being perceived to 'be good/healthy', and now make decisions based on what feels good or bad in my body and listen to and learn from my inner expert. Beyond food, it has changed my relationship with myself and my friends and family. It has gifted me with more compassion for myself and others in a real and lasting way. I tended to make decisions around food based on so many external and social cues, and I have learned to put myself first when I really need to.

The most important piece of advice I could give you is to dive straight into it. Don't wait to commit to doing the one-to-one work. Stick to it and give it time. Don't be disheartened by how long it might take. Constantly remind yourself to approach your experiences with curiosity and not judgement – I needed reminders of this plenty of times. External support from Niamh was game-changing for me, and the benefits to your life are well worth the work and the time. It's never too early or too late to start this journey – just start it.

Emma

'You just need to take a chance and believe in yourself.'

I was utterly exhausted from years of dieting and restrictive eating when I started my intuitive eating journey. It was very challenging at first learning to trust my body, listen to what it needed, and feel my feelings after years of squashing them down. As I progressed on my intuitive eating journey, working one to one with Niamh, reading books on intuitive eating and diet culture, and changing my social media feed to see that bodies can come in all different shapes and sizes, I slowly retrained my way of thinking. I went from years of speaking badly to myself to learning to accept myself for who I am, and I now have self-compassion and self-worth, valuing myself for who I am in the here and now.

A significant difference that intuitive eating has made in my life is the way in which I now deal with social situations. Previously I would have been so anxious, wondering if I was taking up too much space or how I would cope if there was food involved in the gathering. In the past, I ate nothing or watched what everybody else was eating to ensure I wasn't overeating! Now, if there is food at an event, I eat foods that satisfy me and don't worry at all about what anybody else is doing or if they are watching me.

Eating has become more about what I need to fuel my body but also what I need to feel satisfied. When I started with Niamh, my eating was irregular, and I felt like I was no longer interested in food. I slowly started cooking meals for myself again based on what I felt like, what my body needed, and what made me feel satisfied after eating. Over time this connection to my needs became stronger, and now I eat a wide variety of foods. It has become incredibly important to me to listen to what my body is asking for to feel satisfied.

For anybody reading this who is thinking of embarking on their intuitive eating journey, I know it can be hard to trust your body and to let go of restricting some foods you may have been denying yourself for years. I know because I've been there, and I understand the fear of 'if I start eating that food, I won't stop', but you will. You just need to take a chance and believe in yourself. Trust that you will one day learn how to listen to your body again instead of listening to society telling you what to do with your body. And also, throw away the scales. Your worth is about so much more than a number on the scales.

Conclusion

Things to Remember

Ever since I was little, I've loved to read (bookshops were and still are one of my favourite places), and when I reached my late teens, my book of choice moved from fiction to non-fiction. There is so much incredible information to absorb from a personal development book. Sometimes when I read these books myself, I feel overwhelmed, put them back on the bookshelf, and, sadly, never implement the learnings. I always said that if I ever wrote a book, I would add a section at the end summarizing the key points discussed in each chapter to help remind readers of the high-level learnings from the book. Yes, these are the things I think about — I know, I'm a true nerd (and proud)! Thus I've dedicated this final section to summarizing each chapter so that, as you are on your journey towards food freedom, you can flick back and remind yourself of the key 'things to remember' from each chapter.

At the end of every session with my clients, I ask them about their key takeaways, and sometimes they are different to what

I expected. I always approach every client with an attitude of collaboration: we are a team. I am the expert of the process, but I'm not the expert of you. When I work with people, either in a one-to-one capacity or through any of my online programmes, it's like a coming together of two experts. I want to do this with you too, dear reader. As you have read through this book, you may have had different insights to those I have listed as the key 'things to remember' from each chapter, which is why I have left some empty lines to write down your own key takeaways. Think about it like your very own therapy session with me! There are no rules about how to answer this, but the below prompts might help you decide what takeaways you could add to this section:

- ☐ How did you feel reading the chapter?

- ☐ Did it bring up any emotions, insights, or memories for you?

- ☐ Did you have a physical reaction to the content discussed?

- ☐ Was there a particular sentence or section that resonated with you?

- ☐ Did you have any lightbulb moments?

- ☐ Is there one action step you'd like to take after reading the chapter?

Part 1: REMOVE

Remove what you've learnt from diet culture that keeps you stuck in a place of food stress and obsession and hinders your health and growth as a human being.

Chapter 1: Deconstructing Diet Culture

- ☐ Diets do not result in long-term weight loss.

- ☐ We do not currently have any safe and effective methods for long-term, sustainable weight loss.

- ☐ Uncovering and rejecting diet culture in your internal and external world is a possible and necessary first step towards rebuilding a healthy relationship with food and body image.

My key takeaways

_____

_____

_____

_____

_____

Chapter 2: Detaching from Appearance Ideals

- ☐ The widespread nature of body image struggles in our society is rooted in diet-culture messaging and contributes heavily to an unhealthy relation-ship with food. Rejecting these oppressive appearance ideals is an important part of the process.

☐ Rebuilding a positive body image will help to protect a healthy relationship with food.

☐ Everybody can benefit from body image work regardless of size, shape, or age.

My key takeaways

_____

_____

_____

_____

_____

Chapter 3: The Power of Permission

☐ Food restrictions must be removed to feel in control around all foods.

☐ There is no such thing as 'good' or 'bad' foods.

☐ We need to embrace an abundance rather than a scarcity mindset around food or else the deprivation effect, i.e. overeating, will persist.

My key takeaways

_____

_____

_____

_____

_____

Chapter 4: Uncovering the Inner Critic

☐ Your inner critic will wreak havoc if it's allowed to take the wheel and drive the bus.

☐ Self-compassion and developing an inner friend are the antidotes to the inner critic.

☐ We must challenge faulty food beliefs that uphold the inner critic and lead to guilt and shame surrounding food.

My key takeaways

Part 2: RECONNECT

Reconnect with the needs of your mind and body to give you the information that you need to begin nourishing yourself with ease.

Chapter 5: Reconnecting with the Self

☐ Your inner expert is a wise guide who knows what you need at any given moment.

☐ You hold all the wisdom within about what, when,

and how much to eat, along with what else you need to meet your other needs.

☐ Mindfulness is the key to reconnecting with your inner expert.

My key takeaways

_____

_____

_____

_____

Chapter 6: Reconnecting with Hunger

☐ Honouring your hunger cues and eating regularly will protect you from uncontrolled overeating.

☐ Connecting with your hunger cues will help you assess how much food you need and when.

☐ There are four types of hunger, all of which are valid reasons to eat — we eat for more than just physical hunger.

My key takeaways

_____

_____

_____

_____

_____

Chapter 7: Reconnecting with Satisfaction

☐ Connecting with your satisfaction cues will help you assess what food you need to feel satisfied.

☐ Mindful eating will help you to become reconnected with your satisfaction cues.

☐ There are two parts to satisfaction — taste and body satisfaction — that help to merge pleasure and health.

My key takeaways

_____

_____

_____

_____

_____

Chapter 8: Reconnecting with Fullness

☐ Fullness sorts itself out for the most part when the other concepts within the 'remove' and 'reconnect' stages are worked through.

☐ Stopping eating at comfortable fullness takes time and practice and will not be possible without honouring the other concepts of intuitive eating.

☐ Removing the obstacles to feeling your fullness will help you stop eating when you are comfortably full.

My key takeaways

_____

_____

_____

_____

_____

Chapter 9: Reconnecting with Emotions

☐ Emotional eating is not inherently bad; we all do it from time to time. It only becomes an issue when food becomes our default or only coping mechanism.

☐ Reconnecting with your emotions will help you to understand the messages they are giving you and to subsequently meet the needs that food is filling.

☐ Expanding your coping-skills toolkit will not only help with emotional overeating but will also help you to get through life in general.

My key takeaways

_____

_____

_____

_____

_____

Part 3: RE-ESTABLISH

Re-establish health-promoting behaviours from this new perspective that you've developed by first removing anything that does not serve you and then reconnecting with the needs of your mind and body.

Chapter 10: Sleep

☐ Sleep is possibly one of the most important but underrated aspects of health and well-being.

☐ Good sleep starts with your daily habits.

☐ Creating a sleep ritual or routine that sets you up for a good night's sleep can be incredibly supportive if you struggle with this.

My key takeaways

_____

_____

_____

_____

_____

Chapter 11: Self-Care

☐ Self-care is health care.

☐ Self-care is so much more than bubble baths, trips

away, or getting your nails done. The most important elements of self-care cannot be bought.

☐ Self-care is not always beautiful and requires you to act in ways that support your future self.

My key takeaways

_____

_____

_____

_____

_____

Chapter 12: Stress Management

☐ Unmanaged stress is a silent destroyer and will wreak havoc on your health if not managed.

☐ Nervous-system regulation plays a role in your long-term health and how you feel on a day-to-day basis.

☐ There are two steps to managing your stress levels:
      Step 1: Notice your symptoms of stress
      Step 2: Employ a stress management strategy

My key takeaways

_____

_____

_____

_____

_____

Chapter 13: Food and Nutrition

☐ Eating for general health and well-being doesn't need to be that complicated.

☐ Gentle nutrition is a flexible, non-diet, and evidence-based approach to healthy eating, one that centres on you and your unique, individual needs.

☐ To uncover your unique nutritional needs, pay attention to how food makes you feel.

My key takeaways

_____

_____

_____

_____

_____

Chapter 14: Movement

☐ Intuitive movement is about finding joy in activity and letting your body guide you to what suits you best on any given day, week, month, season, or year.

☐ Movement should be fun and joyful; if it's not, it's a sign you need to change things up.

☐ Everything counts: doing some physical activity is better than none.

My key takeaways

_____

_____

_____

_____

_____

Having the Strength to Move Forward

To experience transformation in your relationship with food, you will need to make changes. Some of these changes may feel challenging, but transformation doesn't happen without challenge. Transformation happens when you begin to change things in your life you once believed you never could. True strength comes from doing hard things, not doing things you already know how to do. When you begin to take steps towards change, you will most likely meet resistance. This resistance is a sign that you are growing and moving closer to the transformation you seek. The brain is resistant to change because it requires unfamiliarity. To the brain, anything that is unfamiliar is unsafe. With change, you are literally carving new pathways in the brain. When we expect resistance, it can help us lean into it when it arises.

The journey towards food freedom is not always linear and you may come up against obstacles in your path. Know that these are there to teach you something. They are a sign that something else needs to be healed. Look at them with curiosity instead of judgement. Approach them all with loving kindness and compassion. What message are they trying to give you? The journey to true food and body image freedom is a radical one. It will ask you to challenge and opt out of certain belief systems you may have always believed were true. Some people in your life may still hold these belief systems and they may not understand the path you've chosen. This is normal for any transformation we go through in life – the people we love don't always go through the same transformation as us at the same time.

You may fall along the way. You may get pulled back into dieting or into the oppressive beliefs that uphold it. See this as an indicator of how deeply embedded diet culture is in our society, rather than an individual failure. Opting out of diet culture in a world obsessed with thinness is radical, but it comes with so much freedom. Know that If you fall at any stage, you can pick yourself back up again and return to where you left off without judgement. Write down every single little win that you experience along the way so you can remind yourself of them when things get hard.

Rebuilding your relationship with food and finding food freedom truly is transformational. I have been privileged enough to witness this transformation first-hand in many of the clients I have worked with. It is not an exaggeration to say that I have seen lives changed as a result of taking that first step into intuitive eating and staying on the path, and I have heard the phrase 'this is life-changing' from my clients many times. Food has been the entry point for greater transformation for many of my clients. Many of them found it hard to believe that transformation was possible at the beginning of their journey, but they decided it was harder to stay where they were than to take the steps towards change. Many of these people achieved what they set out to achieve through their courage, bravery, and unrelenting persistence. Many of them now live a freer and happier life as a result. They look back at how far they've come and thank that part of themselves that believed change was possible.

I know you can do it too. All you need to do is take that first step, and if you've made it to the end of this book, you've done that. You are now on the path towards food freedom. Rather than thinking about all the steps you need to take to get there, simply focus on taking the next step. Before you know it, you will find yourself getting closer and closer to the transformation you seek. Every step counts. I'm rooting for you.

Final Words

This book is about liberation. It's about freeing yourself from the constraints that society has conditioned you to believe you must abide by to belong. These cultural constraints encourage us to feel apologetic for who we are if we do not fit the box that's been created for us, impacting our relationship with food, body, and self. As an antidote to this message, this book invites you to consider the possibility of showing up as your authentic self with *no apologies*. Because no one should have to apologize for who they are, how their appearance changes over time, or what size or shape body they inhabit.

There aren't many words I've read that align with this message more than those of Donna Ashworth. So much so that I'm going to end this part of our journey together with one of her inspirational poems. I hope her words inspire you as much as they continue to inspire me.

Wave The White Flag

There are many choices available to us women in this life —
but when it comes to your body, there are only two:
Accept it
Or don't.
You see, if you choose to accept your body, you will soon
start to love it, admire it, look after it.
These things all follow in the wake of your acceptance.

When you realise that this vessel for your soul, for your
spirit, is an instrument of such high design and fine tuning
that it boggles the mind to even think about, you will enter
into a phase which I like to call 'peace, at last'.

You will care nothing of spare fat, grey hairs, loose skin.
You will realise, eventually, that the body's purpose is not to
look good, to attract friends, partners, successes — that it
is, in fact, your spirit which does all of those things.
If you would only allow it to shine through and work its magic.

Your body, my friends, has but one job, to see you safely
through this adventure of life, to allow your spirit to reach
its potential.
That is it.
If you are on the path of not accepting your body — you are
in for a very long battle — against an enemy you have no
power to defeat. Nature, time, biology, fate . . .

You don't have the weapons to fight those powers.

Wave the white flag.
Give in.
Accept.
It is then that your life will truly begin.

— *Donna Ashworth*

Resources

Online Resources

All of the resources that have been mentioned throughout the book can be found online on my website nutritionwithniamh.com.

- 'Do You Have a Healthy Relationship with Food?' Quiz and Training Video
- The Ireland and UK Intuitive Eating and Anti-Diet Facebook Group
- 'Observing Your Thoughts' Meditation
- 'Compassionate Friend' Meditation
- 'Inner Expert' Meditation
- 'Chocolate' Meditation
- 'Progressive Muscle Relaxation' Meditation

Further Reading

If you'd like to do some further reading around the area of non-diet nutrition, body image, yoga, movement, and other health-related topics, then consider picking up the following books.

- Tribole, Evelyn, and Resch, Elyse, *Intuitive Eating: A Revolutionary Anti-Diet Approach* (Essentials: 2020)
- Tribole, Evelyn, and Resch, Elyse, *The Intuitive Eating Workbook: Ten Principles for Nourishing a Healthy Relationship with Food* (New Harbinger: 2017)
- Harrison, Christy, *Anti-Diet: Reclaim Your Time, Money, Well-Being and Happiness Through Intuitive Eating* (Hachette UK: 2019)

- Johnson, Anita, *Eating in the Light of the Moon: How Women Can Transform Their Relationship with Food through Myths, Metaphors and Storytelling* (Gurze Books: 2000)
- Rye, Tally, *Train Happy: An Intuitive Exercise Plan for Every Body* (Pavilion Books: 2020)
- Klein, Melanie, and Guest-Jelly, Anna, *Yoga and Body Image: 25 Personal Stories About Beauty, Bravery, and Loving Your Body* (Llewelyn Publications: 2014)
- Emanuela, Victoria, and Metz, Caitlin, *My Body, My Home: A Radical Guide to Resilience and Belonging* (Hardie Grant Books: 2020)
- Sobczak, Connie, *Embody: Learning to Love Your Unique Body* (And Quiet That Critical Voice!) (Gurze Books: 2014)
- Kinavey, Hilary, and Sturtevant, Dana, *Reclaiming Body Trust: A Path to Healing and Liberation* (TarcherPerigree: 2020)
- Kite, Lindsay, and Kite, Lexie, *More Than A Body: Your Body Is an Instrument, Not an Ornament* (Harvest: 2020)
- McBride, Hillary, *The Wisdom of Your Body: Find Healing, Wholeness and Connection through Embodied Living* (Brazos Pres: 2021)
- Neff, Kristin, *Self-Compassion: The Proven Power of Being Kind to Yourself* (Hodder and Stoughton: 2011)
- Saunt, Rosie, and West, Helen, *Is Butter a Carb? Unpicking Fact From Fiction in the World of Nutrition* (Piatkus: 2019)
- Hartley, Rachel, *Gentle Nutrition: A Non-Diet Approach to Healthy Eating* (Victory Belt: 2021)
- Strings, Sabrina, *Fearing the Black Body: The Racial Origins of Fat Phobia* (NYU Press: 2019)

- Gordon, Aubrey, *What We Don't About When We Talk About Fat* (Beacon Press: 2020)

Further Listening

There are loads of amazing podcasts about intuitive eating, body image and debunking diet culture: I only wish I could list them all! These are my favourite ones.

- The Binge Eating Dietician Podcast by Jo Moscalu
- Intuitive Eating Ireland by Sinéad Crowe
- Maintenance Phase by Aubrey Gordon and Michael Hobbes
- Body Image with Bri by Brianna Campos

Endnotes

Introduction

1. Wansink, Brian, and Sobal, Jeffrey, 'Mindless eating: The 200 daily food decisions we overlook', *Environment and Behavior*: January 2007
2. University of North Carolina at Chapel Hill, 'Three Out Of Four American Women Have Disordered Eating, Survey Suggests', *ScienceDaily*, 23 April 2008
3. Satter, Ellyn, 'What is Normal Eating?', Ellyn Satter Institute, 2018
4. 'What is Disordered Eating?', Academy of Nutrition and Dietetics, 28 February 2020
5. Anderson, James, et al., 'Long-term weight-loss maintenance. a meta-analysis of US studies', *The American Journal of Clinical Nutrition*: 1 November 2001

Chapter 1: Deconstructing Diet Culture

1. Harrison, Christy, *Anti Diet: Reclaim Your Time, Money, Well-Being and Happiness Through Intuitive Eating* (Hachette: 2019)
2. Harrison, Christy, *Anti-Diet: Reclaim Your Time, Money, Well-Being, and Happiness through Intuitive Eating* (Hachette UK: 2019)
3. Calogero, Rachel, et al., 'The impact of Western beauty ideals

on the lives of women: A sociocultural perspective', *The Body Beautiful* (Palgrave Macmillan: 2007)

4. Harrison, Christy, *Anti-Diet: Reclaim Your Time, Money, Well-Being and Happiness Through Intuitive Eating* (Hachette UK: 2019)

5. Harrison, Christy, *Anti-Diet: Reclaim Your Time, Money, Well-Being, and Happiness through Intuitive Eating* (Hachette UK: 2019)

6. Strings, Sabrina, *Fearing the Black Body: The Racial Origins of Fat Phobia* (NYU Press: 2019)

7. Lelwica, Michelle, *The Religion of Thinness: Satisfying the Spiritual Hungers behind Women's Obsession with Food and Weight* (Gurze Books: 2010)

8. Harrison, Christy, *Anti-Diet: Reclaim Your Time, Money, Well-Being and Happiness Through Intuitive Eating* (Hachette UK: 2019)

9. Fothergill, Erin, et al., 'Persistent metabolic adaptation 6 years after "The Biggest Loser" competition', *Obesity* 24(8) (Silver Spring): 24 August 2016

10. Keys, Ancel, et al., *The Biology of Human Starvation* Vol. II (University of Minnesota Press: 1950)

11. Bacon, Linda, and Aphramor, Lucy, 'Weight Science: Evaluating the Evidence for a Paradigm Shift', *Nutrition Journal* 10(9) (American Society for Nutrition): 24 January 2011

12. Stunkard, Albert, et al., 'The Body-Mass Index of Twins Who Have Been Reared Apart', *The New England Journal of Medicine* 322(1483–1487) (Massachusetts Medical Society): 24 May 1990

13. Stunkard, Albert, and McLaren-Hume, Mavis, 'The results of treatment for obesity: a review of the literature and report of a series', *A.M.A. Archives of Internal Medicine*, 103(1) January 1959

14. Fildes, Alison, et al., 'Probability of an Obese Person Attaining Normal Body Weight: Cohort Study Using Electronic Health Records', *American Journal of Public Health* 105(9) September 2015

15. Dansinger, Michael, et al., 'Meta-analysis: the effect of dietary counseling for weight loss', *Annals of Internal Medicine*, 147(1) 3 July 2007
16. Nordmo, Morten, et al., "The challenge of keeping it off, a descriptive systematic review of high-quality, follow-up studies of obesity treatments', *Obesity Reviews: an official journal of the International Association for the Study of Obesity* 21(1) 21 January 2020
17. Tomiyama, Janet, et al., 'Long-term effects of dieting: Is weight loss related to health?', *Social and Personality Psychology Compass*, 7(12) (Wiley: 2 December 2013)
18. Foster Wallace, David, *This is Water: Some thoughts, delivered on a significant occasion, about living a compassionate life* (Hachette UK: 2009)
19. Kabat-Zinn, Jon, *Wherever you go, there you are: Mindfulness meditation in everyday life* (Hachette Books: 1994)

Chapter 2: Detaching From Appearance Ideals

1. Kite, Lexie, and Kite, Lindsay, *More Than A Body: Your Body is an Instrument, not an Ornament* (Harvest: 2020)
2. McBride, Hillary, *The Wisdom of Your Body: Finding Healing, Wholeness, and Connection Through Embodied Living* (Brazos Press: 2021)
3. Schilder, Paul, *The Image and the Appearance of the Human Body* (Routledge: 2013)
4. Wood-Barcalow, Nicole, et al., *Positive Body Image Workbook: A Clinical and Self-Improvement Guide* (Cambridge University Press: 2021)
5. Pearson, Adria, *Acceptance and Commitment Therapy for Body Image Dissatisfaction: A Practioner's Guide to Using Mindfulness, Acceptance, and Values-Based Behavior Change Strategies* (New Harbinger Publications: 2010)
6. Runfola, Cristan, et al., 'Body dissatisfaction in women across

the lifespan: results of the UNC-SELF and Gender and Body Image (GABI) studies', *European eating disorders review: the Journal of the Eating Disorders Association* 21(1) January 2013.

7. Kearney-Cooke, Anna, and Tieger, Diane, 'Body Image Disturbance and the Development of Eating Disorders' *The Wiley Handbook of Eating Disorders* (Wiley-Blackwell: 2015)

8. Bennett, Kate, and Stevens, Robin, 'Weight Anxiety in Older Women', *European Eating Disorders Review* 4(1) March 1996

9. Jackson, Kathryn, et al., 'Body image satisfaction and depression in midlife women: the Study of Women's Health Across the Nation (SWAN)', *Arch Women's Mental Health* 17(3) 13 March 2014

10. Robertson, MacKenzie, et al., 'Exploring changes in body image, eating and exercise during the COVID-19 lockdown: A UK Survey' *Appetite* 1(159) 1 April 2021

11. Frederick, David, 'The swimsuit issue: Correlates of body image in a sample of 52,677 heterosexual adults', *Body Image* 3(4) 3 December 2006

12. Kelly, Colette, et al., 'Weight concerns among adolescent boys', *Public Health Nutrition* 19(3) 19 February 2016

Chapter 3: The Power of Permission

1. Epstein, Leonard, et al., 'Long-term habituation to food in obese and nonobese women', *The American Journal of Clinical Nutrition* 94(2) August 2011

Chapter 4: Uncovering the Inner Critic

1. Singer, Michael, *The Untethered Soul: The Journey Beyond Yourself* (New Harbinger Publications: 2007)

2. Neff, Kristen, *Self Compassion: The Proven Power of Being Kind to Yourself* (Hodder and Stoughton: 2011)

Chapter 5: Reconnecting with the Self

1. Khalsa, Sahib, et al., 'Interoception and Mental Health: A Roadmap', *Biological Psychiatry: Cognitive Neuroscience and Neuroimagining* 3(6) June 2018
2. Tribole, Evelyn, and Resch, Elyse, *Intuitive Eating: A Revolutionary Anti-Diet Approach* (Essentials: 2020)

Chapter 6: Reconnecting with Hunger

1. Tribole, Evelyn, and Resch, Elyse, *Intuitive Eating: A Revolutionary Anti-Diet Approach* (Essentials: 2020)

Chapter 7: Reconnecting with Satisfaction

1. 'The Principles of Mindful Eating', *The Centre for Mindful Eating*, January 2016
2. Thomas, Laura, *Just Eat It: How intuitive eating can help you get your shit together around food* (Boxtree: 2018)

Chapter 9: Reconnecting with Your Emotions

1. Tribole, Evelyn, *The Intuitive Eating Workbook. Ten Principles for Nourishing a Healthy Relationship with Food* (New Harbinger: 2017)
2. Johnston, Anita, *Eating in the Light of the Moon: how women can transform their relationships with food through myths, metaphors and storytelling* (Gurze Books: 2000)

Chapter 10: Sleep

1. Hirshkowitz, Max, et al., 'National Sleep Foundation's updated sleep duration recommendations: final report', *Sleep Health* 1(4) December 2015
2. Del Gallo, Federico, et al., 'The reciprocal link between sleep and

immune responses', *Archives Italiennes de Biologie* 152(2-3) June–September 2014

3. Cappuccio Francesco, et al.,'Quantity and quality of sleep and incidence of type 2 diabetes: a systematic review and meta-analysis', *Diabetes Care* 33(2) February 2010

4. Walker, Matthew, *Why We Sleep: Unlocking the Power of Sleep and Dreams* (Simon & Schuster: 2017)

Chapter 11: Self-Care

1. Reading, Suzy, *Self-Care for Tough Times: How to heal in times of anxiety, loss and change* (Aster: 2020)

Chapter 12: Stress-Management

1. Davis, Martha, and McKay, Matthew, *The Relaxation & Stress Reducation Workbook* (New Harbinger Publications: 2008)

2. Wickens, Andrew, *Foundations of Biopsychology* (Prentice Hall: 2004)

Chapter 13: Gentle Nutrition

1. Hartley, Rachael, *Gentle Nutrition: A Non-Diet Approach to Healthy Eating* (Victory Belt Publishing: 2021)

2. Knuppel, Anika, et al., 'Meat intake and cancer risk: prospective analyses in UK Biobank', *International Journal of Epidemiology* 49(5) 1 October 2020

3. Reuter, Simone, et al., 'Oxidative stress, inflammation, and cancer: How are they linked?' *Free Radical Biology and Medicine* 49(11) 1 December 2010

Acknowledgements

Many people, and not just the name on the cover, have gone into the publication of this book. It takes a village! I have to start by thanking the entire team at Harper Collins Ireland, who made this book a reality. To Catherine Gough, for introducing me to the world of publishing and keeping me at ease from the beginning. To Conor Nagle, who kept me grounded when I was flailing and never let the first-time author jitters pull me off track. And to my editor Flora Moreau, for always being in my corner and understanding the vision from the off. Thank you for believing in me, even when I didn't believe in myself. To anyone else who worked on this book, you helped make a dream come true.

To all the practitioners, trailblazers and activists I have learned from who have crafted the non-diet movement, thank you for your work and emotional labour. I am always learning from you all and am deeply grateful. Without you and your work, I wouldn't be able to do the work I do today.

For all my incredible clients — your experiences have shaped the contents of this book, and it's a privilege to walk alongside you while you rebuild your relationship with food and your body. Your faces came to mind when I was reaching for inspiration to fill these pages. Thank you for trusting me with your stories and allowing me to be your tour guide. You teach me something every day and make me into a better practitioner.

I care deeply about each one of you and wish for you to live your life unapologetically, as you deserve.

To anyone who has followed, liked, shared or commented on my content on social media, listened to my podcast or supported me in any way by sharing my work with others, thank you. It really does mean a lot and keeps me going, especially when I feel like no one is listening. You have been an essential part of getting the message out there that health is possible, no matter your body size and in turn, are a crucial part of the social shift of liberation for all bodies.

To my amazing friends and family — thank you for always supporting me, just as Niamh, the person, when I truly needed it. Sinéad Crowe and Jo Moscalu were always on hand for panicked voice notes, content checks and last minute phone-calls. Thanks for having my back, both personally and professionally. Many of my friends listened to me rant and provided me with encouraging words when I needed them. I appreciate every message of encouragement and each one of you. And to my dearest friend Laura Burke - thank you for being my rock throughout this process. For all of the visionary conversations, rants and excited dances around the kitchen. You bring light and safety to my life and are one of the most supportive people I know. I couldn't have done this without you. And to my parents, whom I know without a doubt are always there for me, cheering me on from the sidelines. You have made me into the person I am today and have been instrumental in getting me to where I am. This book would not exist without either of you and the unwavering love and encouragement you've given me my whole life (even with all my crazy ideas). I love you all.